LOST
ARROWS

LOST ARROWS

COPING *with the* DEATH OF A CHILD

S. E. HUFFAKER

Scott Huffaker
Info@lostarrowsbook.com
www.lostarrowsbook.com

Lost Arrows, Scott Huffaker —1st ed. ISBN 979-8985288001

CONTENTS

IN MEMORY OF OUR

Beloved Dylan

Sweet Judy Booth

Reese Johnson

and Stephen Grimes

APPRECIATION PAGE

There are so many people that I could include on this page, because so many blessed us through the years in regard to Dylan. If I tried to list everyone I know I would surely miss a lot of folks and I don't want to do that. Everyone is deeply appreciated that was involved in our lives through the years. So I am only going to list those that were closely engaged after Dylan's death and while I wrote this book. I still may miss someone and if I do, please forgive me but know you were appreciated.

First, I have to thank Tammy, my wife and children Joseph and Lucy who have daily patience with me. I am deeply thankful to my children Lena and Tyler for reuniting me with Dylan. I am thankful for my parents Robert and Wilma Huffaker who have stuck by me through thick and thin.

Secondly, I am thankful for my friends Robert Reid, Tyler Gillespie, Christina Broom, Nancy Hudson, Jason Brand and Jonathan Wontz who almost daily were supporting me and encouraging me.

Thirdly, I am thankful for our dear friends Angel and Brian Lamar who walked the path with us.

Fourthly, I am thankful for Austin Hardison for allowing us to assist with Red Mountain Grace in memory of Dylan. And for Connie Bowen one of Dylan's nurses for directing me their way.

I am very thankful for my great friend Tyler Gilreath who helped me with this book. And finally, I am very thankful for Steve Gordon, Brittany Liebert and Steve's team in helping bring this book to fruition!

May God bless you all richly!

INTRODUCTION

It was shortly after 10, on the morning of August 6th, 2021. I had just dropped Joseph, my youngest son, off at his work. I had just crossed the bridge into Florida on Highway 98, headed to work in Pensacola.

Unexpectedly, I received a call from Lena, my oldest daughter. She frantically asked was I driving and if so, I needed to pull over! I knew in my heart, before the words rang out, what she was about to say.

As I pulled over and stopped, she said "I'm sorry, I'm so sorry. Dylan is dead!"

She further stated that the police were at Poppy's house (where Dylan lived) and that Poppy (their maternal grandfather) was all out of sorts. She said that I needed to get to Bay Minette as soon as possible!

He was gone…

Fast forward to the evening of September 27th, 2021. My wife Tammy and I were watching the second episode in the newest season of NCIS, ironically titled "Nearly Departed." Jethro Gibbs (played by Mark Harmon) and Tobias Fornell (played by Joe Spano) were newly reunited in a truck on a stakeout for a serial killer. A portion of their conversation went as follows:

(Gibbs) Been a few weeks. How you doing?

(Tobias) Good, real good actually!

(Gibbs) You still doing that group thing of Palmer's?

(Tobias) That group thing is a revelation! You got to come to the next meeting. Counseling has done wonders for me! And, uh, it could for you, too...

After a rant of chastising Gibbs for burying himself in his work, Tobias continues...

(Tobias) How long will it take for you to fill the void inside you?

(Gibbs) What void?

(Tobias) We all have voids my friend. You know, Gibbs you and I we're like twins. We've both lost jobs. We've both lost wives. More than one. And now I've joined your club by losing a kid.

(Gibbs) That's not a club!

(Tobias) It's not a club I would ever sign up for. What would they even call it? I mean, you lose your parents, they call you an orphan. You lose your spouse they call you a widow, but...

You lose a child there is nothing to call you. There is no word for it! That's how bad it is!

When I heard this, I knew this had to change! I know and have known many parents who have lost children, but even so I have dreaded it for the past 32 years, because I knew it was a very potential reality for Dylan to die before me. I never dreamed of the depth, breadth and width of the pain I would experience. I knew something had to change. There had to be a way to define, uplift and include in society a group of people who probably experience more emotional pain, by losing a child, than anyone in this life.

The first thing that came to my mind was what King David said in his Psalm 127,

³ Children are a heritage of the LORD: and the fruit of the womb is his reward.

⁴ As arrows are in the hand of a mighty man: so are children of the youth.

⁵ Happy is the man that hath his quiver full of them...

I believe, as a parent, our children very much define us. So as a defining term I deemed that losing a child was like losing an arrow that one cannot ever find in this life again.

An arrow held great value in times past and took much labor to bring to perfection, to one day release into the world on its own.

LOST ARROW

An arrow was born this day
a tedious and rewarding task
still much work to be done
to prepare for the day
that it enters the air on its own
work for the straight and narrow
it's closer to becoming an arrow
a notch is added
for proper grounding
fletching for proper flight
a pointed tip
so it may stick to the task
now it goes to the air
training is in session
success and joy
are its rewards
many days bring satisfaction
one day the air
is in its wings
its destination
cannot be seen
now a lost arrow.

By S.E. Huffaker

We parents who have lost children, would all agree that the pain is overwhelming. *But there is a way to cope.* Having a background in banking and sales for the last 40 years, I have assisted tens of thousands of people in managing their decisions about their finances, families and businesses. In this book we will provide some practical ways to cope with what sometimes seems overwhelmingly daunting.

As a side note, this book is not a venture for making money. This is strictly for philanthropic purposes, which I will talk about in Chapter 1. Join me on this journey as we learn to cope in a more productive way and help others and ourselves in the process!

PREFACE

What Should I Expect?

It was the middle of July 19th, 2021, to be specific. It was hot and crowded in Destin, Florida. I had a meeting to go to this particular day. I wasn't expecting anything out of the box, but little did I know that what I was going to hear this day would change, in a positive way, my frame of mind and thought processes forever.

The speaker was a former Israeli sniper who retired and entered the business world. He had been very successful in building huge sales teams and pushing them to their limits. The topic he would share this day was on NLP (Neuro Linguistic Programming). This was not a foreign topic to me as I had read a couple of Tony Robbins books and that is the premise of much of his material. But what this speaker said was so profound to me that since this day my way of thinking has been forever changed. What he said this day that I am going to share may sound simple, yet if you let it sink in and embrace it, I fully believe you will understand why it has had such a profound effect on me.

"Beliefs Are Feelings. I Mean Beliefs Are Just Feelings!"

What did he mean? As soon as he said it, my mind began to spin. I knew he was right on point. You might be asking, why would this be so moving for me (the author) or you the reader? Let me share. As people, as humans, our beliefs and what we embrace originate from many places. What we are taught, typically comes from people we believe, like (or love) and trust (parents, grandparents, etc.). Our beliefs come from our education system. Our beliefs come from our experiences. This or that happens so this must be the way things are. For many, beliefs come from media and officials. We embrace things and believe things that we feel comfortable with or are easy for us to embrace. We believe things that come from our friends or the community, organization or church we are involved in. We believe things that may come from "religious" authorities. Our beliefs (feelings in their infancy) can originate from many different sources and avenues. And these beliefs were mentally and emotionally birthed as feelings.

You still may be asking what does this have to do with grief?

Hang with me a few more moments and I will shed light on the path you are following me down. In one of his books, Tony Robbins likened beliefs and convictions to a tabletop with legs. A belief is merely the top of the table. But as one gathers more evidence and or affirmations concerning that belief the legs start to attach to the table and create a conviction.

And *here* is where we have to be irrefutably honest with ourselves...

With whatever we believe (matured feelings and possibly a conviction) did we *personally* do the necessary due diligence to verify *whatever* we believe, is the *ultimate irrefutable* truth?

So how does this all connect? This book is going to share and explore grief from a very diverse perspective, as if we were in a spaceship looking down on earth. There are many things that have helped me, and I believe will help you cope and learn to cope better. And frankly it may require a more open mind than you have had up to this point.

This book is not intended to be a "faith" based book and there will be times when different religious sources and materials will be quoted and used. As a caveat, I personally profess my beliefs as a Christian, and I know not everyone does, so I come humbly and respectfully with a desire and heart to help anyone and everyone who wants to migrate to a higher level—no matter one's beliefs.

This perspective, that I will share, has helped me become a more merciful, loving, caring and non-judgmental individual. All these improved attributes have helped in my healing and coping process.

Now that this discussion is out of the way, here is what you can expect. For many reasons, I believe everyone needs to share their story about themselves and their child or children they have lost. So in the first chapter I will share Dylan's story, *our* story. Next, we will explore how different cultures, peoples, populations and religions approach grief. Some of this material will be historical in basis.

Then the subsequent chapters will be specific things we can embrace and do to migrate to a better place of coping. Then finally as the saying goes if you fail to plan, you plan to fail. So the finale will be an outline and plan to help us reach a higher plane of coping. Thank you for choosing to join me in this path thus far and I look forward to sharing more toward our mutual healing, coping and helping throughout the rest of the book.

CHAPTER 1

Robert Dylan Huffaker—Is This What It Feels Like To Have A Firstborn Son?

An ancient story goes like this: A slave travels with his master to Baghdad. Early one morning, while milling through the marketplace, the slave sees Death in human form. Death gives him a threatening look. The slave recoils in terror, convinced that Death intends to take him that day. The slave runs to his master and says, "Help me. I have seen Death, and his threatening look tells me he intends to take my life this very day.

I must escape him. Please, master, let me leave now and flee on camel so that by tonight I can reach Samara, where Death cannot find me." His master agrees, and the terrified servant rides like the wind for the fifteen-hour journey to Samara. A few hours later, the master sees Death among the throngs in Baghdad. He boldly approaches Death and asks him, "Why did you give my servant a threatening look?" "That was not a threatening look," Death replies. "That was a look of surprise. You see, I was amazed to see your servant today in Baghdad, for I have an appointment with him tonight in Samara." - *Money, Possessions & Eternity, Tyndale Press 2011*

No one can escape death...

When a child is born, typically we are not focused on the fact that one day they will die. We are enthusiastic and enthralled with all that they are (and will be) and all the joy that will come. I couldn't say that with Dylan. Although excited about my firstborn son, I was overwhelmed with fear about his future demise. Within a few days of his birth, I knew deep down that his life would not be normal. I always believed that he wouldn't live past the age of 12 or so.

Let me rewind to the past for a moment. As far back as I can remember, I always wanted children. I always loved playing with the kids and babies at church and everywhere I went. When I was 12 my nephew Michael was born and within a few days later my niece Amy was born. I was happier than a pig in the mud. Those are some of my best memories— being around them, babysitting them. My brother Stanley (Michael's dad) and his wife Patricia came over for lunch after church almost every Sunday. After Michael was born, later Melissa, those Sundays were truly the high points in my week. We didn't see my oldest brother Steve or Amy very often, as they lived in south Alabama and we lived near the Tennessee line in northwest Alabama, yet I was always anxious to get to see them and play and love on them.

Fast forward to 1983...

When I married Donna, my oldest children's mom, she already had a daughter. Lena was a very sweet, quiet child and never truly a bit of trouble. But even to a 19-year-old who loved children, at that time in my life it wasn't the same as having a child who was your own flesh and blood.

To say that our relationship (Donna and me) was anything less than a constant storm would be an understatement. Unfortunately, there are few times that I can recall that I had any peace about our relationship. Yet still we plunged through it. We got married in January of 1983, divorced in August of 1985 and then got back together in March or April of 1986. On March 1, 1987, our first child Kymber was born. Oh, such a happy day for me! But similar to Dylan she had some heart issues as well. When she was about six months old, she was diagnosed with SIDS (Sudden Infant Death Syndrome) and we had to put her on a heart monitor for 18 months. As her heart rate got low in the night, the monitor would alert us and we would have to wake her to get her heart back to normal status. To say the least this was exhausting, not only from lack of sleep, but from again facing the fear of death of a child I loved so dearly, my firstborn. Prior to Kymber's birth, my good friends Barry and Melinda Grimes lost their 2-year-old son. This only escalated my deepest fears.

In my mind, the stage was set...

On March 6th, 1989, our beloved Dylan was born. Due to the health problems that Kymber had experienced, we had gone to USA Children's & Women's Hospital in Mobile to deliver. Prior to his birth, his health issues had not been identified. So shortly after his birth and the nurses flurrying around, we were taken aback in complete surprise.

They called in a specialist, a pediatric cardiologist, Dr. David Mayer, and this is what he shared. Dylan's heart was upside down and on the wrong side. He had tricuspid atresia, which is where there are three chambers in the heart versus the normal four. He had pulmonary stenosis, which was partial blockage of his artery to the lungs, and he also had a hole in the top of his heart. I was in a daze, and I was facing my greatest fears. The potential of losing a child.

The hospital visits, the heart caths (cardiac catheterizations), the tests went on endlessly. After a bit of time, I truly can't remember how long it was until we received a prognosis. They had consulted with the doctors at the University of Alabama at Birmingham (UAB Hospital), specifically Dr. James K. Kirklin and Dr. Albert D. Pacifico and the best they felt they could offer was a procedure when Dylan turned three, known as a Fontan procedure. They would go in and rework the heart makeup as best as possible and that would give him a few years. They believed that he could live a guarded life with meds and care for a few years. Per Dr. Kirklin, Dylan was not a candidate for a heart transplant.

Donna and I were emotional wrecks. I had not been close to my family since Donna and I had gotten married and had not really darkened the door of a church more than a handful of times since I moved to South Alabama in 1982. I had gone a few times to Fairhope Church of Christ but I wasn't engaged. That was about to change.

Lena, Kymber and I started attending regularly and the church and the people there were very comforting, loving and prayerful for Dylan, our family and his situation. Dylan was constantly being prayed for. This being part of a church, a community, was key to maintaining our path and sanity. We had a support system in place.

Fast forward to 1992...

These three years went by rather quickly. Dylan was loved and cared for by his sisters and in the meantime, Dylan had a new baby brother, Christian Tyler. He was born On November 15, 1990. Thankfully Tyler wasn't born with any health issues.

We had found a couple that kept children, Bill and Patsy Schuler and Donna had started a cleaning business, so the children began staying with them during the day as Lena went to school and we worked. I had been working at GMAC and had progressed rather well, but they wanted me to move from Mobile to be promoted and I didn't believe I could do that given Dylan's condition. His doctors were familiar with his situation and we had believed in their abilities—that they were his best medical solution providers. So I had to make a job change, and that was scary due to the insurance scenario and knowing what we were facing in just a few months.

I started working at Grady Buick/BMW as a Finance Manager. Don, Gary and Kelly Grady were very gracious and understanding of our situation and supported us 100%. This was in March of 1992. We were surrounded with overwhelming support from friends, family, church friends. My former bandmates helped with entertainment for a benefit: Terry Goins, Jack Smith, Bill Menas and Barry Grimes. Barry had lost a child (Stephen) in previous years to a quick onset of spinal meningitis. In retrospect not sure how he was able to play that with us. Also, a good friend from church, Phillip Brown, who helped in raising several thousand dollars to assist with the anticipated expenses. We were surrounded with love and care.

In April of 1992, Dylan went to UAB to have the Fontan procedure. This went fairly well initially. Dr. Pacifico performed the surgery and the results achieved were as well as could be expected. They felt that Dylan should have some good years in front of him. However, suddenly, things took a turn for the worse. Water began filling up in his pericardial sac (the membrane around the heart). They rushed him into surgery again and removed the sac from around the heart. For several days things were touch and go and they we were not sure if he was going to make it.

I'll never forget during this time the band I was playing with (Michael Garrahy and Celebration, https://www.mfgent.biz/music-and-band-photos) as a part time gig. We had just played an event at the Officers Club at Naval Air Station Pensacola. I was driving back home knowing Dylan wasn't faring well and as I passed the rest area at the Florida/Alabama line I prayed with great sorrow. I prayed, *"God please don't take my son, take me if someone must die but please don't take him"*. For the first time ever, I realized I loved someone more than myself.

As miraculously as miracles come on this earth, the next morning Dylan began to improve and within about a month he was back home and we were together as a family again. Dylan was thriving and doing well. So many prayers were prayed and answered on his behalf. In my mind Dylan was the closest I had experienced to a miracle in this life.

When Dylan was five, the Make-A-Wish Foundation, as they do with many, granted Dylan's wish for us to go to Disney World. We had a great time and he got to see his hero, Mickey Mouse. It was a wonderful time and we created memories we will all cherish. Things rocked along for several years. Dylan and his siblings did the normal things—went to school and had a rather normal life.

In the fall of 1999, Donna filed for divorce. I could write an entire book on all that transpired over the years after this, but I am going to keep it simple and focus on the segment that Dylan played throughout this time. I will say there were many things that happened that seemed horrible at the time, that I learned from them, and that I see (in retrospect) that their happening was a benefit to me down the road. The divorce process lasted a little over a year and during this time we each had the children for a week at a time. This same process was settled on and continued after the divorce.

It was specifically on September 11, 2000, that Tammy (now my wife) and I first connected online. Within a couple of weeks we decided to have lunch and went to Mikee's Seafood in Gulf Shores. She wasn't sure about going to lunch with an older man; she was 22 and I was 38. But Kay Norton, an old friend, worked at Myer Real Estate with Tammy and she assured her I was an okay guy. My divorce was final in October of 2000, but although we talked frequently, Tammy and I didn't start dating until January of 2001.

Tammy had had her own cross to bear as her father was killed in a tragic accident, right after her high school graduation. She had encountered this dreaded event of death. As with most of us it was extremely hard for her to deal with it. More on this in a moment...

Tammy and I married on October 23, 2001. She wasn't sure how well she was going to deal with three half-grown children and the whole blended family scenario. But September 11th had just happened, and I think much of the world had the mindset that life is short and we must capitalize on "the moments."

Within weeks we were back in court (Donna's favorite pastime). This was the beginning of many battles that continued until her death.

Fast forward to 2003...

Due to the nature of the accident of Tammy's father's death, she, her mom and her sister received an insurance settlement. Tammy decided she wanted a big house, so her mom gave her a couple of acres next to where she lived and we began the planning stages of building a new home. She wanted the kids to have their own rooms. So the plans ended up being for a three-story seven-bedroom home. Looking at it from the road many people thought it was a *bank building*, due to the height and design. In retrospect, although I'm thankful, too many times the wish to dial back time and use better wisdom and go smaller has been felt and expressed.

This new house angered Donna to new heights and she was done having shared custody of the children. To say I was an emotional basket case would be a grave understatement. Facing the thought of having my children ripped away from me, especially for no good reason other than more money was hard to take at the time.

I will reiterate here that the lessons and experiences I encountered through the next years, although painful and taxing, only prepared me for *the now*. Over the next years I got thrown in jail countless times over false allegations and "contempt"—again, all with money being at the root of the actions. It was never about the true best interest of the children. I didn't see Dylan from that July 2004 until he graduated from high school in 2009. And that was only briefly—for maybe an hour.

In April of 2010 Dylan was admitted into the hospital at UAB. This was a short time after his 21st birthday. The Fontan procedure had lasted as long as it was going to. Dylan was going downhill fast. On August 14th I got a call while I was at a customer's house and I don't even remember now who called. But I was told that Dylan had had a successful heart transplant. I was beside myself in emotions.

You may remember from an earlier chapter that Dr. Kirklin, who performed the Fontan procedure when Dylan was three, had told us that Dylan was not a candidate for a heart transplant.

How ironic is it that the doctor who performed Dylan's heart transplant was Dr. Kirklin's son! He was the first in the world to do a heart transplant on anyone with the many abnormalities Dylan had.

Once again, this showed me and the world the closest thing I believe I will ever witness as a *miracle* in this life.

Donna made many attempts always to have me falsely thrown in jail. She was regularly trying to get me to come see Dylan. I had cut off all contact with her due to her continued escapades.

About a month after the transplant I was able to go see him. This time was no different, *but I knew what to do.* I took about ten people with me and when once again she tried to cause a scene in the ICU and have me thrown in jail. I humbly bowed out.

I only got to see Dylan momentarily—not even talk—as he was unconscious. Dylan continued to improve and in December of 2010 Dylan and his mom moved back to Bay Minette to live with Donna's father.

It wasn't long until Donna and I were in court again. Yet, after all these years I had learned how to maneuver and manage this game. We went to court one more time in 2014. After that I began representing myself. That experience was very enlightening and eye opening about the inner workings of the family court system. It wasn't a win but it was a "keep things at bay" strategy. Frankly that was the best I could hope for and I was thankful for the reprieve, even though it infuriated many (and I mean *many*) people.

Still no seeing Dylan through 2016. Tyler was doing well and he was living in California. Tammy and I had been blessed in 2005 and 2007 via *in vitro* with two wonderful children, Joseph and Lucy. I had many things to be thankful for. But as any parent would and will, I still missed my oldest son and missed being a part of his (what I knew deep down) *shortened* life.

In November, 2016, things had changed in the political arena and I highly suspected my "keep at bay" move might soon fall apart. I had taken Joseph to see Casting Crowns, a Christian rock band, perform. I personally hadn't listened to them much but Joseph had and he wanted to go see them.

I was very moved. What was the most moving was when Mark Hall (a youth pastor and the band's lead vocalist) told the story of how he came to write the song "Just Be Held." I could 100% relate. I knew that was all I could do—let God hold me in his arms.

Admittedly I was at one of my lowest points during this time. On the afternoon of December 18, 2016, Tyler called me. I was completely not expecting what he was about to share. Their mom, Donna, had passed away that morning. Things were about to change!

Personally, I felt relieved and blessed from my lone perspective. Hopefully now all the warring and court appearances were over. Yet because I love my children, if I had held the power to bring her back I would have. It was unbearable to see my children suffer over the loss of their mom. After a few days, with comforting as best I could from a distance, they buried their mom.

Lena and I continued to talk on occasion over the years, but she had become disenchanted with me over some things that transpired on her wedding day (December 18, 2019). But there was an event that happened while she was a teenager where I was supportive and her mom wasn't and she had greatly appreciated my response at that time. Thankfully I had done something right with her and for her. For this reason and with her being the great young woman she had become, she spearheaded an effort to reunite me with Dylan.

Dylan had been led to believe that I didn't care for him, that I didn't love him and that I didn't want anything to do with him. It was a glorious, joyful and wonderful day when Lena and her family brought Dylan to me and we all had breakfast together. My heart was so happy! It took a few days but even through his grief Dylan began to relearn that I was the loving father he had grown up with as a child.

Over the next few years we became closer than we ever had been. We loved each other and I was *so* thankful. We did things together—go to his doctor visits in Birmingham, spend Christmas with Mom, Dad, and my family, see movies, and do all the other things that Dylan liked to do. These cherished memories will stay with me forever.

At the beginning of 2021, Dylan began having some respiratory problems. They got worse. He had gone to his local doctor but didn't seem to get better. So we scheduled him a visit with his doctors at UAB. Tyler actually flew back to meet us and go to Birmingham.

That was somewhat of a fun trip, just me and my older sons. Something that we had not gotten to do in a long time—just us being together. But Dylan was insistent that he was dying, and yet all the results from his heart and lung tests were good. He had a little congestion, so they gave him some antibiotics to help clear it up. This was in February and for a bit he seemed to improve. Yet in June we were back there again— same good results as far as his heart but some congestion that they continued to treat with antibiotics.

In the middle of July, he had become worse *again* and he checked himself into the hospital in Fairhope, Alabama. With all the Covid goings on, I couldn't visit him in the hospital. We talked daily and the doctors had gone into his lungs and scraped the congestion.

He was doing better. He stayed in the hospital until the 31st, when he was discharged. I continued to talk to him via phone and he was doing well.

The night of August the 4th was the last time I got to speak to him. I called to check on him and he was still feeling good. We spoke for a moment and talked about getting together soon to go do something. We told each other we loved each other and we hung up.

Lena spoke to him the next night. He had just gone to sit in his living room and said that he was getting stuffy, but said that he was feeling good. He went to bed and never awoke. His death is still somewhat of a mystery, yet I chose not to dig into what the cause was as I knew that wasn't going to bring him back and felt it would only create more pain and not comfort.

I wanted to create a memorial for Dylan, so I called Connie, his nurse at UAB and asked her did she have any thoughts of worthy causes that needed donations. She shared with me about an organization called Red Mountain Grace in Birmingham. They assist with families that have to come to UAB or other hospitals in the area for an extended stay.

We fully understood this dilemma. So I felt this would be a worthy cause to assist with and direct gifts to (and monies otherwise spent for flowers). Thus far, as of the writing of this book, a little over $7,500 has been raised. My plan is to direct 40–50 % of the net proceeds of the sale of this book and journal toward that cause. The remaining monies will be used to market the book and to establish physical and virtual groups for those within the lost children community.

Thank you for continuing with me down this journey. Next, we will explore how others outside our "circle of beliefs" deal with grief and mourning. See you in the next chapter!

CHAPTER 2

I Thought Division Was A Mathematical Operation

Division among peoples, races, beliefs (spiritual and secular) and nations has always been a part of reality on this earth. Has it always been as ever-present as it is today or have there been times in history where the flavor was milder? The reason I pose the question is because I believe you would agree, many times this division stops us dead in our tracks in considering other ideas, thought processes and resolutions that may well benefit us far better than what we have on our present agenda. I want to share with you this following bit of history to demonstrate the influence, magnitude and monumental effects that *division* can cause and has caused.

The Concept Of "Race" A Recent Development

The etymology of the word "race," as used in regard to people, can be traced only to the sixteenth century. Around 1500 the English word race carried the sense of a group with a common occupation; by the 1540s the word had evolved to refer to a generation of people; and it wasn't till about 1560, that it was used to denote a tribe, nation or people of common ancestry. Race's modern meaning, "one of the great divisions of mankind based on physical peculiarities" is from 1774.

The modern emergence of racism and preoccupation with racial identities can thus be located sometime after the Middle Ages, developing through the Age of Exploration and becoming fully established in the colonial era.

Taken from "The Myth of Equality: Uncovering the Roots of Injustice and Privilege," by Ken Wytsma (2017, published by InterVarsity Press, Downers Grove, IL. www.ivpress.com)

This is a true and real picture of how beliefs evolve from feelings. As history will tell us, certain races began to be viewed as little more than animals. Slaves were imported into America by the droves. Unfortunately, the *feeling* of superiority of one race over another set its hooks in the future of what is present today. This evolved into the belief of racial discrimination. And now that we have this on the forefront of our minds, let's delve (with an open and unprejudiced mind) into how others around the world and throughout history have dealt with and coped with grief and mourning.

Throughout time, even though mourning and grief rituals vary, there is one sentiment that seems consistent... No one wants to die, even with the promise of an afterlife. That sentiment is very well spoken in Hamlet, Shakespeare's famous play:

The undiscovered country from whose bourn
No traveler returns, puzzles the will
And makes us rather bear those ills we have
Than fly to others that we know not of?

Hamlet – III, i.79-82

Land Of The Lost Rituals

Before we explore different cultures, I believe it is important to note that the west lost much of its grief culture at the time of the Plague and moving forward. So many people died, and people were fearful of having anything to do with the remains as they weren't sure what the cause of the Plague was. This was totally counter to the culture, where mourning the death of a loved one was a big to-do. The plague flooded church graveyards, and many had to be buried in mass graves.

Boccaccio wrote, of Florence 1348 ... "As our city sunk into this affliction and misery, the reverend authority of the law, both divine and human, sunk with it."

Grief, mourning and rituals began to evolve....

Life is sometimes like a map: in order to determine where we are and where we must go, we must look at where we have been.

French historian Philippe Ariès (July 21, 1914 – February 8.1984) delved deeply into the history of death and rituals in his book "The Hour of Our Death." In an article published in the New York Times on Feb 22, 1981, Robert Nisbet does an excellent job of summarizing what Mr. Ariès discovered.

> MAN is the only species to bury his dead. Of the recurrent crises of the human condition - birth, marriage and death - it is death that has generated the largest number of rituals, most of them based on a belief in an afterlife. It is as though an instinctive disposition exists in man to reject the thought of death as definitive, as the completion of the life cycle. Whether we leave food, clothing and implements in the burial place - as people have as far back as the Paleolithic Age - or simply offer prayers at graveside, the premise is the same: The community that nourished in life must also nourish in death. Death takes place within the community; death is a wound to the community; death is a departure from the community. That is a fair way of epitomizing the significance that death has had in all the great world religions.

It is also a fair way of describing Philippe Ariès' view of the way death was experienced up to two centuries ago, when significant counterforces began to operate in the West. For many thousands of years, death, funerary and mourning rites were not very different in the West from those that had existed everywhere in human society; the power of the community was unchallenged in matters of death as well as birth and marriage. But in our century, Mr. Ariès argues, there has been an "abdication of the community" from death. Death is left to an "enormous mass of atomized individuals." Death has become an increasing solitary, almost "invisible" phenomenon."

We were well into the 20th century and funerals were still being managed in the home, in the United States and Europe. Many times the funeral, its style, and embellished deathbed rituals were planned out ahead even by the person who was dying.

As mentioned previously, the Death arena began to change at this time in history. The medical community with its advances began to extend their control over death. The funeral industry began the takeover of the management of the dead. And then what emerged was a greater fear over death and the dead body. Death was no longer familiar, as it had been in times past. Now it was and is threatening and horrific. In today's society we have a plethora of horror movies and ghosts. How could we expect any less of how we feel?

Grief became and is a compacted process!

After we highlight what different cultures and peoples do to mourn and cope with grief, in this and the next chapter, we will summarize what items, processes and healthy rituals may be of assistance to us in the coping and grieving process.

Tombs, Pyramids & Celebration

In past decades, probably the most prominent ancient culture to come to mind is that of the ancient Egyptians.

Let's explore some of the things they did and find the value that they provide us with today.

First, their perception and embrace of death was different than many. In Egypt, death was not the end of life, but the beginning of the second leg of one's journey. No word in ancient Egypt correlated with the concept of "death" as no longer being alive. It was just a transition of sorts. Once the soul successfully passed the judgment of Osiris, it went on to the eternal paradise of the Field of Reeds.

Herodotus (b. c. 484-425 BCE, d. c. 413 BCE), wrote of Egyptian rites and what they did to mourn. This is what he wrote:

> As regards mourning and funerals, when a distinguished man dies, all the women of the household plaster their heads and faces with mud, then, leaving the body indoors, perambulate the town with the dead man's relatives, their dresses fastened with a girdle, and beat their bared breasts. The men too, for their part, follow the same procedure, wearing a girdle and beating themselves like the women. The ceremony over, they take the body to be mummified. (Nardo, 110)

There is a lot of rich history from Egypt about all the procedures, rituals and practices surrounding not only death but the preparation for the burial, and the sendoff to the afterlife. It was a several-month process to prepare these items, even for the poor.

The Egyptians celebrated life by means of their tombs. They also had mortuary cults provide offerings to their souls in perpetuity. Gratitude was first and foremost in the lives of Egyptians. They believed that ingratitude was the gateway sin to let all other sins into one's life. Therefore, they were grateful for all that life had to offer and what they enjoyed in the "present life" phase.

The Egyptians celebrated life and death throughout the year. It was a daily occurrence. There were no temple days—just worshipping the gods and celebrating daily. However, they did have special occasions or festivals to focus on different aspects of their religion and culture. There were several celebratory seasons but there was one in particular that celebrated the souls of those who had passed on. It was called the Wag festival.

The Wag Festival was usually celebrated immediately after the Wepent-Repent Festival, but the date was later changed to mid-August due to the lunar calendar. It is one of the oldest festivals in ancient Egypt and has been in existence since the unification of upper and lower Egypt.

The festival was celebrated to mark the death of Osiris and the journey of those deceased to the underworld. Ancient Egyptians celebrated the Wag Festival by making paper boats and floating them on the Nile from east to west, which was believed to flow into the afterlife. Paper shrines are also made and floated on the Nile for the same reason. People also honored the dead by carrying food to their tombs and offering it to them. The celebration was led and performed by the priest belonging to the temple of Osiris, or Anubis.

Interestingly enough there is a strong correlation between this festival and the Day of the Dead, celebrated on another continent thousands of miles away.

Day Of The Dead And The Aztec Connection

If you are familiar with the Day of the Dead (Dia de Los Muertos), you would normally think of Halloween paired with November 1 and 2. However this is a misnomer. This festival dates back to the Aztec empire and is rich in cultural history. Prior to Cortez and 1519 the Aztec community in southern Mexico and central America was a cultural epicenter. A couple of sources shared varying dates with one source stating that it was celebrated at the beginning of our month of August and continuing throughout the entire month. Another source stated that the festival started in July and lasted throughout the month of August. In both cases the first month or days (and this coincides with the current Day of the Dead celebration) was for the souls of children and the second portion or day for adults. November 1st is deemed as "Day of the Angels" or "Day of Innocents," with November 2nd being the day the souls of adults are remembered and celebrated.

At the root of the beliefs of the celebration is that the dead return to our world from the afterlife during this time. Most celebrating the Day of the Dead honor these returning spirits with altars, shrines and gifts. Many go and visit the graves during this time. It is also during this celebration that death-centric iconography has a leading role. Death themed decorations, performances about death, dressing up as skeletons along with buying and selling of skeleton figurines are part of this celebratory process. The dead are honored and the visual reminder of our very sure mortality is presented.

Kuru Japan

When I think of the Japanese, I think of a very respectful people, a very honorable, hardworking and intense group of people. Once again demonstrating beliefs and feelings, this same sentiment was not held by those who fought in World War II and their contemporaries. But yet, their death ceremonies and grief rituals are of the same pattern of respect and honor. They follow the auspices of two different religions, Buddhism and Shinto. Ninety percent of all Japanese funerals are a blend of Buddhist and Shinto traditions. Most Japanese homes have both a Buddhist altar and a Shinto shrine.

It is their belief that in order the keep the spirits of the dead out, when a household member dies, both the altar and shrine are closed and covered. Then, next to the bed of the deceased, a small table with simplistic flowers, candle and incense are placed to honor the dead.

And then, there are 20 steps the Japanese follow:

1. "Matsugo no mizu," the washing of the lips. A close relative wets the lips of the deceased, giving the body its last taste of water. This is to be performed as close to the time of death as is possible.

2. The "yukan," the washing of the corpse. Several family members may be involved in this practical and ceremonial washing.
3. "Kiyu hokoku," the announcement of the death. The family announces the death to the spirit world through prayer and memorialization at the family shrine.
4. "Makura naoshi no gi." The phrase means "pillow decorations" and the ritual involves placing the deceased in such a way that the head is propped up on a pillow, facing north. Offerings of food are to be made to the gods at this time. A sword or knife is placed by the side of the deceased.
5. "Nokan no gi," the placement of the dead body of the deceased in a coffin.
6. "Kyuzen nikku," or daily food offerings to the deceased. These food offerings are to be made twice a day until the body is given its final resting place. Traditionally the favorite meals of the deceased are prepared.
7. "Ubusuna jinja ni kiyu hokokuh," the announcement of the return of the spirit to the local shrine.
8. "Bosho batsujo no gi," the earth purification ceremony. The priests from the local shrine will purify the ground to be used for the grave site with water and prayer.
9. "Kessai," when the priest purifies himself in preparation for the funeral. This normally occurs through ceremonial washings and prayer.
10. "Tsuya sai," this is considered the wake. Mourners gather to express condolences to the family and present their offerings to the gods, the shrine and sometimes the family.
11. "Senrei sai," which means the transfer of the spirit. The priest transfers the deceased's spirit from the

body into a wooden tablet. The tablet is held over the body of the deceased while the priest offers ceremonial prayers.

12. "Settai", which is a word for refreshments. Food that has been prepared at a different location to prevent the contamination of death is served to the mourners. This food may be anything from a light snack to a substantial meal.

13. "Shinsosai", the funeral service. The room where the funeral will be held is purified, prayers and offerings are made to the gods, and eulogies honoring the deceased are given by the priests.

14. "Kokobetsu shiki", the farewell ceremony. Mourners leave the funeral by walking, single file, past the deceased. The mourner is to say final goodbyes to the deceased and offer prayers and word condolences to the family.

15. "Hakkyu sai no gi" is the departure of the coffin. The coffin is prepared for travel to the grave site. A sword is placed on the coffin and banners are placed around it so that the deceased becomes aware that it is time to move on.

16. "Soretsu", is the funeral procession that transports the coffin to the cemetery or crematorium.

17. "Hakkyu-go batsujo nogi", the home where the funeral ceremony has taken place is purified. In addition, the funeral altar is removed and a new altar is set up inside the house.

18. "Maisosai", is the offering of burial rites. Family and close friends will gather at either the grave site or crematorium with the body. Offerings are made on

behalf of the deceased and are placed with the coffin. Prayers are led by the priests.

19. "Kotsuage," means the picking up of the bones. Bones are removed from the crematorium ash and are placed in a vase.

20. "Kika sai" and means coming home. Ashes that are not buried are brought to the home and placed in the family shrine. The bereaved offers thanks to the people who have participated in the funeral. Prayers and offerings are given on behalf of the deceased.

The family of the deceased will then be in a period of mourning for 49 days. Once a week they will visit the grave to place fresh flowers and to burn incense. On the 3rd, 7th and 49th days, they will have a short memorial service at the site, led by the Shinto priest. During these 49 days, the family cannot participate in any form of celebration or entertainment. (https://eterneva.com/blog/death-rituals/)

Russia And Krásnyj Úgol

I've always thought of Russia as a superpower, a huge nation that has always been a longstanding enemy/friend of the United States. And one where poverty was prevalent and people were at the mercy of the "State."

A few years back when I bought my sailboat, I started taking lessons from Lanier Sailing in Pensacola. It was a group class and lasted for several days spread out over a course of weeks. One of the couples were from Russia. He was from Pensacola but had moved to Russia many years before. He had been the

CFO for a major oil exploration company. He had married a Russian lady and they had moved back to the states to retire.

We became good friends and when they found out I had a sailboat they wanted to come with me to try it out. A couple of months after our classes had ended, we did just that. We went out into beautiful Pensacola Bay and took her for a sail. What I learned that day really wasn't surprising yet like so many other things I had begun to discover in recent years I discovered that not all that is shared in the mainstream is on point. Russia through their eyes and experiences was a beautiful place and still a land of opportunity. They were very much like us and us like them.

To some extent their funeral traditions are very similar to ours, except they still have a piece of history that is from olden times. Many Orthodox Russians practice what is called Krásnyj úgol, meaning the "red, shining or beautiful corner." It is a corner in a room that is iconic, where pictures of saints, candles and crosses are displayed.

By tradition, the head of the deceased backs up to this iconic corner. The body is laid out here for three days. Prior to being laid here the body is washed, dressed and typically dressed in white with a belt. They will have a formal funeral service typically at one of their Russian Orthodox churches and a meal afterwards where the family and friends of the deceased gather.

They do have commemoration times at the 3rd, 9th and 40th days, which are very important for them to remember their loved ones. A towel and a cup of water are placed on the window sill for the soul of the deceased to revisit to wash and have a rest. Many in Russia believe the soul wanders for 40 days prior to proceeding to the afterlife. Anniversaries and half anniversaries of the death are commemorated by the bereaved by praying, giving alms to the poor and eating Kolyva, a dish made with wheat berries and served at memorials.

China—The Other Superpower

When I first read about what I'm going to share, I had to wonder where it originated. More on that later. The traditional mourning period, called 守喪 (shǒusāng) is one year. The mourning period for the first-born son can last up to three years, though *modern Chinese families observe a period of 49 days*. During that time, the family prays for their loved one every week.

In Hong Kong, China, where many of the old ways have been somewhat protected from the political climate, there are many temples used for honoring ancestors. The deceased are always being venerated. Prayers are said and conversations are had with their deceased loved ones. Yet one of the most prominent practices is that of burning joss paper (incense scented paper in the shape of coins) many times. The deceased are treated very much like gods, as some have said there is really no difference in the minds of many Chinese people in regard to the gods and their ancestors. This will shortly lead us to the subject of veneration and where it originated.

Various Other Cultures And Peoples

On the island of Bali, the Balinese do not mourn. In their culture this is one of the biggest events of *celebration and gaiety*. They believe that celebrating is their utmost responsibility as they cremate their dead because they are fulfilling sacred duty by liberating the souls of the dead.

The Filipinos still use some of the traditions that were in America prior to the 20th century. The body remains in the home in a casket and there is a wake for 3–9 days. All during this time someone must stay with the body and sleep in the room with the body. A prayer is said at 7:30 pm to ward off evil spirits. Candles are lit and must stay lit for 40 days. One sect of the Filipinos, the Apayao, bury their dead under the kitchen. (Stay tuned for the origin of this practice.)

Jewish Practices Concreted In History

Jewish funeral and mourning rites date back some 5,000 years. One of the first mentions of their periods of grief is when Moses died. It is recorded in the book of Deuteronomy, 34:8, in what some call the Pentateuch and the Jews call the Torah. Moses, who had helped free Israel from Egyptian bondage, dies and it is noted that 30 days was the allotted period for mourning. (As a side note both Lena and I experienced a great reprieve of our emotions over the loss of Dylan on the 30th day after his death. And we aren't *per se* Jewish in our practices.)

Current practices still mimic this process. When the loved one first passes the funeral itself is usually completed very expeditiously. The actual preparation and protecting of the one that has passed is managed by the *chevra kadisha*, defined as a formal Jewish burial society. Once preparation is completed, then there's the funeral. Then the 7 days of *hivah* (mourning) begin immediately after the funeral. It is in this time that there is very intense mourning. During this time the family goes nowhere, not even to the synagogue; they don't cook; they do nothing. Members of the synagogue and other friends bring them food. Then the 30 days begins. During this time, they continue to mourn but life goes back to somewhat normal. But there are times of prayer saying what is called *Kaddish*.

> *Exalted and hallowed be His great Name. Throughout the world which He has created according to His Will. May He establish His kingship, bring forth His redemption and hasten the coming of His Moshiach. In your lifetime and in your days and in the lifetime of the entire House of Israel, speedily and soon, and say, Amen.*

> *May His great Name be blessed forever and to all eternity. Blessed and praised, glorified, exalted and extolled, honored, adored and lauded be the Name of the Holy One, blessed be He. Beyond all the blessings, hymns, praises and consolations that are uttered in the world; and say, Amen. May there be abundant peace from heaven, and a good life for us and for all Israel; and say, Amen. He Who makes peace in His heavens,*

may He make peace for us and for all Israel; and say, Amen.

This is said with at least ten people present and it is also said on the anniversary of the loved one's death. Parents are mourned for a period of one year while other family members fall within the 30-day time frame. It is also expected practice to give to a charity or institution in memory of the loved one. This is called *tzedakah*. When the anniversary of the death of the loved one comes again *Kaddish* is said in the synagogue with the lighting of a candle. The flame is representative of the soul. This is called the *Yahrzeit*.

Biblical Preface

As I mentioned in the beginning, it is not my intent to make this a faith-based book, even though I do have great faith in my religious beliefs. I do this to humbly share with anyone that wants to learn and heal somewhat without threat of being spoon fed beliefs. But as I also mentioned I will use the Bible as a historical reference. As a side note, I believe the Bible is separated somewhat into a couple of parts and a subcategory 1. Historical, and 2. Spiritual and as a subpart of Spiritual is Doctrinal. It is in the Doctrinal portion where there is much division. So I humbly ask that you view with me the historical references mentioned throughout the Bible and by other early historians. Through this process we can see where many things originated, what their purpose would have been and ultimately what healthy practices are.

Follow me into the next chapter to see where many of these practices originated and we will correlate these two chapters to determine what can be learned and what is applicable for us in today's world.

CHAPTER 3

Hidden/Erased History—Is There Anything New Under The Sun?

The wise and famous King Solomon said thousands of years ago that there is nothing new under the sun. In this chapter we will find what I believe to be the wisdom of the ancients that Solomon was so famous for and still used today throughout our society. Of wisdom, this illustration has been used:

> "My boy," said the store owner to his new employee, "*wisdom* and integrity are essential to the retail business. By 'integrity' I mean if you promise a customer something, you have got to keep that promise—even if it means we lose money."
>
> "And what," asked the teenager, "is *wisdom*?"
>
> "That," answered the boss, "is not making any stupid promises."

The magnitude, depth, breadth and width of the word "consent" is breathtakingly overwhelming. We make hundreds (or thousands) of decisions every day, and sometimes because of that frequent regularity, we give little consideration to what we have consented to when we make decisions we make. And like the young man above we don't want to consent to any stupid promises. I'll tie this point in momentarily.

As I was writing this book, it so glaringly occurred to me that just as we are once again in a time when history is being erased (I'm not condoning immoral things that happened in history) we not only erase what happened but what potential lessons could be learned from it. From my viewpoint now, I believe that is exactly what has happened to the grieving, mourning, honoring and coping with the death of our loved ones that in times past was more practical—and healing.

So what can we learn from history and the other cultures we discussed? First, much of what is and was practiced originated in ancient times. Join me now as we explore some of those origins and how they can have practical application for us today.

One of the biggest nuggets we can realize and reopen our eyes to is how grief and mourning have been a product of the cancel culture, but much longer ago. We should understand this one simple fact. Prior to 1 A.D. and even shortly after, belief in atheism was basically nonexistent. The vast majority of ALL peoples believed and honored GOD or gods. And they should have, as they were and are ALL real. The vast majority of people and nations also believed in an afterlife.

We don't have the ability to go down that trail and still maintain the focus of this book. However I will provide you some resources at the end of this chapter, so that can you do your own due diligence to determine the truth in this statement about GOD and the gods.

In their book "Veneration" Derek and Sharon Gilbert allude to this cancel culture.

This wasn't just because they lacked modern conveniences, our understanding of the sciences, and access to the Internet, but because they understood that the spirit realm was part of daily life—something we've lost in the modern world, especially in the West. Part and parcel of their reality was interacting with the dead.

As we discussed, the practices embraced by the Egyptians in BCE times and then later the Aztecs, originated from the Amorites and possibly before them in ancient Mesopotamia. They had a monthly ritual called *kipsum* that they used to summon their ancestors to a ritual meal, pouring of water and remembering their name.

This pouring of water many times was facilitated through a libation tube, as many relatives were buried underneath their home floors. They actually used this practice twice a month for their dead kings. If this ritual wasn't used or used consistently they believed it created an unhealthy and unstable spiritual realm. We see those same parallels with the Egyptians, Aztecs and even some of the other cultures have some similarities.

Also of interest is the month of Abu in the Babylonian calendar (the Hebrew month of Ab, or July/August in our calendar) was considered incredibly important in the annual cycle of the *kipsum,* this was the same time as the Egyptian Wag Festival and the original time the Aztecs practiced the Day of the Dead. One purpose of these ceremonies was not only to communicate with the dead but to seek and ask for guidance and prediction of the future.

Thinking of this reminds me of the scene(s) from Silence of the Lambs, with Hannibal Lecter and Clarice batting back and forth with the *quid pro quo.* In other words, give to get. The reason I mention this (and it will fit in momentarily) is because so much of what comes out of Hollywood is "telegraphing." The true message that is being served is far deeper than what it seems on the surface. I was always intrigued by that scene in the movie, but after thinking on this subject of sacrifices and the array of other things that are lifted up for the dead, I have had second thoughts.

This is how dedicated many of the ancient cultures were to the dead and communicating. They would not only provide food sacrifices and honorary services, but also human sacrifices (many times children) and sexual rites. This type of scene was recorded speaking of some of the children of Israel in Numbers 25:1-12. You have to go back to the ancient languages to understand the scope of what was happening as the translations did not do a good job of providing the scope of the event.

To summarize there were many in the camp who were worshipping and offering sacrifices to the dead god Baal-Peor. GOD became jealous and wanted them eliminated. (More on the annihilation reasons later.) So one of the Israelite men brought a Midianite woman to the camp and they began performing a sexual rite in front of Moses and the community of Israel. Then Phinehas, one of the high priests, stabbed them together as they were enjoined in the sexual act.

The ancients were very serious about their communication with the dead and the spirit realm. (And it will make sense shortly as to why I am sharing these things) Yet GOD commanded the Israelites not to do this. I want to share a few things from Dr. Michael Heiser, who has written a plethora of books and material on the ancients and the spiritual realm:

> The law's prohibition against contacting the disembodied (human) dead (Deut 18:11) also provides support for the Old Testament idea of a conscious afterlife. In ancient times it was thought that the dead, as members of the spiritual world, could provide information that was otherwise unobtainable. The Bible prohibits contacting the dead not because doing so was impossible, but because it was possible (1 Sam 28:13); GOD doesn't command people to avoid doing things that are impossible. Rather than seeking insight from the dead, the godly were to seek divine knowledge directly from GOD or through means that GOD had provided, such as the *Urim and Thummim*, the *ephod*, and the *prophets*.

Dr. Heiser further explains their motivation in contacting the dead:

Willfully contacting the other side through means of divination without God's approval telegraphed one's desire to "be like a god," to have the knowledge and attributes of GOD and the other entities that inhabited the disembodied spiritual world.

Here is one other quote from Heiser that will tie in the reason for broaching the subject:

> In Deuteronomy 18:11 we read of one "who inquires of the human dead" (dōrēš el-hammētîm). This description refers to necromancy, contacting the human dead. The fact that this wording diverges from other passages where non-human entities are contacted, illustrates that, as in the wider ancient Near Eastern world, the Old Testament distinguishes ghosts (spirits of human dead) from demonic spirits.

As you can see there is a huge distinction among the entities in the spiritual realm. The problem is we can't see into that side and when we try to contact that side, it's not like a menu at a restaurant where you choose what you want and they bring it to you. You get what you get and you can't pitch a fit. What I am saying is that there are healthy ways and unhealthy ways to interact with our passed-on loved ones and others in the spiritual realm. But more on that momentarily. I want to share a few other examples in this line of thinking before we wrap this chapter up.

In the 1500s there were two gentlemen who were advisors to Queen Elizabeth I. John Dee and Edward Kelley were their names. As a side note many people have a connection in their homes to these two (and they don't even know it). More on that in a moment. They claimed they could speak to angels and created what came to be known as *Enochian Magik*. Many in the occult have used their materials. One such infamous gentleman was Aleister Crowley. If you have watched the television series "Supernatural" you have heard this name. These men were well known for their trying to contact the spirit realm for the *quid pro quo* motive in mind.

Another modern-day example (that is very near and dear to me) of how much we really don't understand how this spirit world works is this story about my dad.

First off, my dad is a 95-year-old minister who still preaches on occasion. He has shared this story through the years. When he was 13, he and his parents lived in northwest Oklahoma in a little town called Afton, which was on the outskirts of Grove, Oklahoma. They were building a lake there—Grand Lake. It's a popular tourist attraction these days. It was manmade and they were going to start filling up the lake.

My dad, his parents and some of his siblings lived across the road from where some of the land was going to be immersed in the lake. My grandfather had cattle on that side of the road where the lake was going to be filling up. So he sent my dad and one of his friends over to drive the cattle back across the road, since their old pasture would soon be under water. So my dad and his friend headed over that way, but before addressing their task at hand they decided to do a little fishing. So they fished for a while, and then my dad decided to head towards the cattle and begin driving them across the road. They were both on horses and my dad left his friend there who promised to join him shortly heading up the cows. Well, when my dad's friend went to meet up with my dad, he was nowhere to be found. He looked all over, so he went to get my grandfather. They continued to look. After looking into the night, they still couldn't find him. So, my grandfather decided to go into Grove and consult a fortune teller.

He did just that and the fortune teller told him he could tell him where my dad was, but he could not accept any money as the process wouldn't work then. He told my grandfather exactly where my dad was and that before he got back across the lake he would be found. About 300 people were searching for him, including the local Boy Scouts. But what's interesting to note is that an elder from a local church actually found him in the exact location the fortune teller said. And because of my mom, whom he hadn't met yet, he would later become a member of that same church where the elder attended.

My dad had been thrown from a horse and knocked out. And what the fortune teller shared is exactly what happened. Even in this we can draw that the fortune teller realized the "rules" and that a *quid pro quo* motive was not appropriate or healthy.

My point is there are things we do not know about the spiritual realm. But just as that fortune teller way back in the1930s knew there were "rules." I also have an acquaintance who is a medium. She says they can connect with the other side through concentration and meditation. There is also another way that some use and that is to channel the spirits from the other side through the medium themselves. She refuses to use that method as she says you never know what spirit and what kind of spirit you may get. They can disguise themselves and their motives.

I also know of many people who have used the infamous Ouija board. (I got your number, L.A. Ha!) They have not had exciting results in that bad things tend to happen when those boards are used. As outlandish as all this may sound there are rules about contact with the Spirit Realm. Some are rules that others adhere to because of their personal experiences and other rules, laws and commandments that were put in place thousands of years ago.

I believe there is a healthier way that we can converse with our lost loved ones, so we have some satisfaction that it is more like a long-distance loving relationship versus "I'm never going to get to talk to you again" feeling.

In his book "The Other Side of Sadness: What the New Science of Bereavement Tells Us About Life After Loss," George A. Bonnano speaks of many people he interviewed who carry on conversations with their lost ones. Sometimes, they do it in special places or they may simply bid them a good morning or good night via their picture. Toward the end of his book, he tells of when he is in China and since he has lost his father in the past he begins conversing with his dad in a one-sided conversation and for the first time feels great peace, joy and some closure.

So, in conclusion of this chapter and this brief study of historical references, I believe there are some things we can add to our routines, practices, etc., that will assist us in our coping with the grieving process in a healthy and comforting way.

1. Consider conversing with your loved ones. Maybe go to a special quiet place that you enjoyed together.
2. Burning candles on special days and special occasions is comforting and helpful. To many the flame represents the soul. I personally keep one lit for Dylan any time I am working at my desk. For me, it provides some peace in knowing that I am remembering him and providing a commemoration for him at my side.
3. When you do have special days (birthdays, holidays, etc.) plan something special on that day in commemoration of your loved one. On the anniversary of their death do this as well. Especially something that you would have enjoyed together.
4. Do things for your loved one as if they were still here in your physical presence. (Not obsessively, but even just in small little things.)
5. Remember that commemoration is an ongoing process.
6. Don't use the *quid pro quo motive* when conversing. Just as relationships in our realm are best when approached with a selfless loving attitude, I believe the same is true when conversing with our loved ones who have passed on.
7. And one final "don't" ... Don't place time frames on your grieving and mourning. Grief was never intended to be compact, convenient and on a time clock.

As I mentioned earlier in the chapter there are several books that will give you a deeper and more comprehensive understanding of the spiritual realm. They will answer many questions about history and even provide insights as to the things that are happening around us today and how they are interconnected. Sometimes I feel like a little kid with a never-ending book of "connect the dots" puzzles. I find new puzzles and nuggets almost daily and you may too. You can continue to connect the dots of the meaning of life and death.

These resources will assist you in connecting the dots. These will not answer all the questions and that is why there are so many books on the subject and why so many continue to be published. I humbly suggest that if you do decide to read them that you do it in the order that I have listed as the books build on each other, almost like the principles of algebra.

1. *"The Unseen Realm,"* by Dr. Michael Heiser
2. *"Reversing* Hermon,*"* by Dr. Michael Heiser
3. *"The Genesis 6 Conspiracy,"* by Gary Wayne
4. *"Gospel Over Gods,"* by Tyler Gilreath
5. *"Veneration,"* by Derek And Sharon Gilbert
6. *"33 Degrees of Deception,"* by Tom C. Mckenney

If you will, follow me into the next two chapters, where we will explore emotions and how they not only play the major role in the grieving process but how we can actually write the script so we can have better outcomes.

CHAPTER 4

Emotional Quicksand— "If I Leave Here Tomorrow, Will You Still Remember Me?"

I wonder if Ronnie Van Zant knew when he wrote those iconic words that one day they would so intensely be associated with his death as well as his life. I have read several stories that stated that he did not believe he would live a full life. Tragically, he left this world at the young age of 29.

I'll never forget that night when the announcement came across the radio airwaves that an airplane carrying the members and crew of the Lynyrd Skynyrd band had crashed in Mississippi. I was lying in bed waiting on my big brother Stanley to get in from work and I heard those crushing words. See, I was going to turn 15 in ten days, and I had begun taking guitar lessons only months before. I was a diehard Lynyrd Skynyrd fan. Also growing up in the Quadtropolis where Freebird was recorded and the fact that Sweet Home Alabama was my new national and state anthem didn't alleviate the deep pit of emotions I felt either.

This connection became even stronger in August of 1993, after Dylan had had his Fontan procedure. As I mentioned, so many people helped us, provided finances, prayed and were just outright kind! Chris Kalifeh, who was one of our external advertising consultants when I worked at Grady Buick/BMW, got Donna and me tickets to see Lynyrd Skynyrd in Biloxi, along with backstage passes to meet the band after the concert. Meeting Ed King, Billy Powell, Gary Rossington and Leon Wilkeson, was a major lifetime highlight for me.

I mention the line "if I leave here, will you still remember me" because I believe very much that at the heart of when someone dies, we almost hear them saying this and we are asking ourselves the same question about them. We are saying to our inner selves *I will never forget you because I love you so much even though you are gone.* And we are asking our inner selves *how much do I need to dwell on and remember you to satisfy my desire to never forget and fulfill how much you would want me to remember you.* And this is only the beginning of the emotional quicksand we begin to encounter.

In the next two chapters I want to cover this emotional gamut we encounter and things we can do to manage these feelings while we are walking our daily walk. When I say "manage," it's not my intent to be insensitive to our feelings but to acknowledge that there are some things we can do so that our emotions don't get the best of us... so we can begin to work toward a fulfilled life even though our loved ones are not with us in this physical realm.

During the time when slave trade was still practiced in some parts of the South, a handsome young man was up for sale. The bids kept rising. Finally, an Englishman gained possession. The young slave began to chide him, "Ha, you buy a slave when slavery has already been abolished in England." The purchaser, however, said, "I have bought you to set you free." The young slave, overcome with emotion, replied, "I will be your willing slave forever."

Just as with the young man in the above illustration, our emotions can turn on a dime. And therefore, I believe the death of a loved one causes an emotional quicksand at times, almost without a way to escape.

In September of this year, Matt Robinson and J Paul Mills, a couple of business mentors of mine, highly recommended I read the book *"Never Split the Difference"* by Chris Voss. They believed it would help me in regard to some business ventures I am involved in.

Chris Voss was an expert FBI hostage negotiator. And his book has been highly acclaimed for teaching how to deal with and understand people, their motives and their emotions. I am so glad that I read it because it was very enlightening when it comes to this subject of managing emotions. Again, I don't use this phrase "managing emotions" with insensitivity, but I realize being able to harness our emotions can by far help us cope and function more effectively.

Especially in Chapter 6 of his book he starts to delve into how to negotiate with those who have taken others hostage. When

I was listening to this (I listen to a lot of books versus reading them, but I also got a hard copy of his book), it resonated with me that when it comes to death we actually become hostages somewhat to our emotions.

One of the first points he makes is that when it comes to negotiating with kidnappers in life and death situations, very little of what is going on is on the surface. In other words emotions are deeply rooted in the equation. A hostage taker's demand is almost always money. And on the surface the family of the hostage believes paying of that ransom will resolve the situation.

And when we grieve we almost have a deep-seated desire *if I can find my "proverbial place" this will get better.* We end up asking all kinds of questions, like why did this happen and what if this would have happened, etc. But just as with a hostage situation there are ways to leverage the emotions and the situation. Many times hostage takers have the mindset that they deserve what they are asking. And frankly many times we believe we deserve better than what the reality is when we have lost a loved one.

The history of hostage negotiations used to hold the belief that compromise was the best solution and splitting the difference would reach a peaceful resolution quickly. Chris Voss realized through his work and frequent encounters that compromise was actually the *worst* solution.

We have this same philosophy in many of our relationships and compromise is embraced to save face and fulfill the feeling that we at least got half of the proverbial cake we wanted. We negotiate and compromise over the premise of fear and to try to avoid the pain.

In the loss of a loved one we have the same feelings. We seek compromise within ourselves, hoping to calm the fears of that loss and to hopefully minimize our pain. And humbly, just as Chris Voss, discovered it was the easy way out and sometimes that's what we tend to migrate to with our emotions. But candidly *that does not work very well.*

Another factor in hostage situations is the deadline. But as Chris found, using that to his favor and learning the motives behind the deadline were key to an effective and peaceful resolution. We do the same, but with us and our emotions our deadline is in the "now" or in the next few minutes. We want a solution. We want to feel better! Are these practices easy? No, but they are the most effective and rewarding!

What Chris also came to know was that in these negotiations, "too few were driven by their actual goals." And in the same way we should have a goal in mind with potential ends in mind—a more peaceful, fulfilled and resolved life, while ever remembering our loved one(s).

So what is a more constructive (and possibly more difficult but actually more accomplishing and rewarding) way to address the hostage taker of our emotions? As the best practices for the most effective hostage negotiation evolved, Chris came to know that there were four questions that had to be answered. These questions needed to be answered so the severity of the threat could be determined. It was when I heard this that I realized this is where our real weakness lies in this emotional quicksand. We tend to ask ourselves the wrong questions in the "hostage negotiations of our heart and mind." Based on these questions and answers we end up many times NOT making the best decisions. And this only thickens the quicksand.

In another quote from Chris' book:

> In "Descartes' Error: Emotion, Reason and the Human Brain," neuroscientist Antonio Damasio explained a groundbreaking discovery he made. Studying people who had damage in the part of the brain where emotions are generated, he found that they all had something peculiar in common: they couldn't make decisions. They could describe what they should do in logical terms, but they found it impossible to make even the simplest choice.

In other words, while we may use logic to reason ourselves toward a decision, the actual decision making is governed by emotion.

So back to the four types of questions and what they are. They are who, what, when and how, and this is what I mean. When we experience the death of a loved one, we tend to ask some of these questions internally and externally (although many of them on the surface are harmless). We typically know the "when" questions. It is the "why" questions that seem to do the most damage and keep us in emotional quicksand longer. There are questions such as:

1. Why did this have to happen to them?
2. Why did this have to happen to me?
3. Why did this happen at all?
4. Why did this happen now?

And so on and so forth... But it is the "what" and "how" questions that we can ask of ourselves that will help us migrate to a better place of coping. Some of those questions would be:

1. How can I honor my loved one today and every day?
2. How can I let them know how much I continue to care and miss them?
3. How would they want me to feel right now?
4. How can I help others in their remembrance?
5. How can I celebrate them on certain days and times of the year?
6. How much time should I and can I spend remembering and commemorating them?
7. What would my loved one want me to be doing right now?
8. What's the best way I can let others know how much I loved them in a positive way?
9. What would my loved one want me to share about them and their life?
10. What would my loved one want me to be doing 3 months, 6 months, or 1 year from now?

What Chris Voss discovered (and we can too) is that these "how" and "what" questions can lead us to a better resolution in what could otherwise be a volatile situation. Focusing on these types of questions rather than those that tend to produce guilt and pain might take some discipline but in the long run we will be better people for it.

Follow me to the next chapter now where we will continue to discuss those things that can help loosen the ties that bind us to the Emotional Quicksand.

CHAPTER 5

Minute By Minute I Keep Holding On

The song, "Minute by Minute," written by Michael McDonald and Lester Abrams, seems to be a song about a guy who feels he is just holding on minute by minute in a breakup that is bound to happen in the very near future. This song won the Doobie Brothers a Grammy nomination in 1980.

It also reminds me of this illustration of a dachshund:

There was a dachshund once so long
He hadn't any notion
How long it took to notify
His tail of an emotion.
And so it happened,
While his eyes were full of woe and sadness,
His little tail went wagging on
Because of previous gladness.

Source Unknown

Both the song lyrics and the poem appropriately and accurately describe many times the emotions we are experiencing and how hard it is to just make it to the next moment. And how we can feel glad and sad in the same moment. It sounds and seems outrageous and it is. But I believe there are ways we can harness our emotions like we spoke about in the last chapter. In this chapter I'm going to share a few other ways that we can bridle our emotions so we can proverbially "keep the horse in the barn until we have it harnessed" and then with confidence we can exit the barn.

To delve deeper into this subject and what remedies are available, first we need to define what emotions are. (I'm sorry, but this is on an elementary level.)

Well as simple as it gets emotions are feelings.

(OH NO, the predecessor of beliefs!) But more on that in a bit. So how do we understand our emotions? Interestingly enough it gets back to one of those really good groups of questions (the "how" questions) in a hostage situation Chris Voss talks about.

1. HOW do I feel?
2. HOW do I know?

There is much written and discussed about the emotions of others and recognizing them, but for purposes of this book we are going to focus on our own emotions. Our ultimate goal is to manage them while still satisfying our need (and our perceived needs of the loved ones we are grieving) to grieve, while trying to ever migrate to a place of functional restoration.

So once we know the answers to the above "how" questions, we also need to dive deeper with a tool called Emotional Intelligence. The term was first coined as you see in this quote:

Peter Salovey and John D. Mayer coined the term "Emotional Intelligence" in 1990 describing it as "A form of social intelligence that involves the ability to monitor one's own and others' feelings and emotions, to discriminate among them, and to use this information to guide one's thinking and action."

Some have further defined the latter part as understanding emotions and regulating emotions. We know that emotions are strongly connected to our memories and experiences (as I mentioned in the preface). If we had a bad experience in the past, our underlying emotional response to the same stimulus will most likely be strong. As I also mentioned in the preface, our emotions are closely linked to our values.

Certain emotional responses could alert us to the fact that our values (beliefs and convictions) have been challenged. When we understand this interconnection between our memories and our values this can provide us with the key to managing our emotional responses. Our emotional responses may have little to do with our current situation or our reasoning, but we can overcome the emotions we need to overcome with reason and being aware of our reactions. I love what Zig Ziglar used to say,

"It's not the situation, but whether we react negative or respond positively to the situation that is important."

— *Zig Ziglar*

So first let's talk a little more about emotional management and then we will dive deeper into emotional intelligence and define their correlation. There has been a lot written and spoken about managing emotions. Aristotle, a Greek Philosopher, said this about managing emotions more than 2400 years ago:

ANYBODY can become angry, that is easy; but to be angry with the right person, and to the right degree, and at the right time, and for the right purpose, and in the right way, that is not within everybody's power, that is not easy.

As he said, it may not be easy, but the question we must ask is, is the extra work—hard work—worth it? Absolutely and emphatically yes! Especially if we want to migrate toward restoration.

So the following is a list of some *positive actions* we can take to manage our emotions:

1. Meditating or praying is very advantageous as it allows you to express in a calm and silent manner what you are thinking or feeling.
2. Exercising is very nurturing as it releases dopamine into the brain, which makes you feel better.

3. Spending some time talking with other people, even if it is what *they* enjoy talking about, as company is always a good healer for the soul.
4. Doing something to distract yourself. When you are experiencing a depth of negative emotions do something to distract yourself. Browsing the internet, reading a book or watching a movie can always serve as a viable distraction.
5. Doing something kind or charitable for other people or charities. We will talk about this in depth in a later chapter, but this is excellent therapy for managing your emotions as it takes your mind off yourself and places importance on others for the moment.
6. Not succumbing to negative thinking. Zig Ziglar called it "stinking thinking." Don't succumb to negative thinking. If you find yourself in its midst search for reasons why the negative perspective is incorrect. Many times this is the product of who we associate with and affiliations we have. Strive (as kindly and humbly as possible) NOT to affiliate yourself with toxic people and toxic situations.
7. Finding the good in what is happening around you. Be mindful and strive to avoid excessive criticism (or any at all) of others or of situations.
8. Spending some time in the outdoors. Fresh air, green grass, or even snow and sunshine can be refreshing, versus staying holed up somewhere.
9. Seeing, noticing, acknowledging the good things in your life. Be grateful for all the good that you have and enjoy. Journaling these thoughts (more on this later) is a good way to focus on your blessings.
10. Doing things that you enjoy and that are good for you.

11. Accepting your emotions... all of them. Embrace your feelings and don't fight them off but learn to politely push through them with grace.

12. Learning to regulate your emotions, not suppress them. Don't sweep them under a rug but be cognizant of them and again use the "respond not react" principles.

13. Magic number 13 requires a bit of an illustration. I can't tell you how many times I have done the following throughout my life. The practice has caused me untold stress and grief. But once I recognized the practice and started striving to not engage in this behavior, Wow! I feel so much better. And my relationships are better. And I am sure a vast majority can somehow relate:

Have you ever been riding down the highway and you pass a police officer or trooper and then in a minute or so you see them in your rearview mirror with their lights flashing and blaring? The first thought that may come to mind is "What did I do? I wasn't speeding" or "I wasn't speeding that much". Your heart is racing, and you have this new unwanted stress. But much to your surprise they scoot around you and pull someone else over. But just for those few seconds we passed judgment on ourselves—maybe minimal but most likely we did while we questioned our integrity.

So, what is the point of the illustration? Let's try our best not to pass judgment on ourselves, situations or anyone. So many times, our judgment is untrue but more importantly unnecessary. It's as if we think it is a protection mechanism, but truly it has the *opposite* effect. When we judge people and situations we create and manifest a persona that many times we have to battle through. Again, an unworthy battle and challenge we don't need. So, #13 is **Strive not to judge people and situations.** Just embrace the moment.

Yes, we can change how we feel. The key to this change is an intense awareness of our emotional responses and what might be behind them. Once we understand these things we can apply some reasoning to our emotions and respond versus reacting. We can ask ourselves some of the following questions to guide us to that port of Emotional Management:

1. How do I feel about my current mindset?
2. What should I do about it?
3. What effects would these thoughts or actions garner for me and those around me, especially my loved ones?
4. Would the action or thoughts I am considering line up with my values?
5. Is there someone else I could ask their thoughts about these things?

These increased levels of awareness are where Emotional Intelligence plays a part. It's almost as if we are on a reconnaissance mission in enemy territory because it may have taken us hostage and we need to find the resolution. So after we may have deliberated over some of the steps above, we can use the following Cognitive Behavior Therapy technique.

It's cleverly named **STOPP**, and it can help improve our Emotional Intelligence. The **STOPP** method can help ground us and feel more in control of our emotions. As with any method of management it may not work all the time and if you feel you need professional help please seek that assistance. I will be providing some resources at the end of the book regarding this subject.

The Five Steps Of Stopp

There are varying versions of this method but the premise is the same.

S – Stop

When negative thoughts or anxiety creep in, or you find yourself with feelings of grief, sadness and loneliness, stop what you're doing. Physically stop. Don't do anything else, don't move. Just stop, wherever you are.

T – Take

Now, take a deep breath. Try a breathing exercise or take deep breaths in through the nose and out through the mouth.

O – Observe

After you have taken some deep breaths it is time to observe what is going on internally, in your mind and what you are feeling. It's observation time. These are some of the things you'll want to pay attention to:

- Your thoughts – What thoughts are going through your mind right now? What are you saying to yourself?

- Your feelings – What emotions are in your mind and experiences?
- Your body – What physical sensations are you feeling? Where are these physical sensations?
- Your behavior – Is there something you are you reacting to? Where is your focus of attention? What are you doing this very moment, in this "now?"

Spend some time observing these things. Don't pass judgment on any of these thoughts and emotions, just take notice that they are there.

P – Pull Back

Pull back to gain perspective and look at the big picture. Here you'll potentially challenge some of your thoughts and feelings from the Observe section. Some of the questions you might ask yourself might be:

- What is another way of viewing this situation?
- Is this thought or feeling a fact or opinion?
- What would I tell someone else who was experiencing these thoughts and feelings?

This challenges negative thoughts and cognitive distortions that can really assist and provide insight before you 'proceed.'

P – Proceed - Practice What Works

Once you have observed your thoughts, feelings, emotions, behavior and even physical sensations, then you can proceed. You will be more mindful of how you feel. Most likely—at least initially—you may find that this changes what you do moving forward. But, if you want to take this a few steps more, then there are some other Ps used by some in the STOPP Technique.

The Extra P's In The Stopp Technique

Different therapists have slightly different techniques when it comes to the STOPP technique. Here are some of the different or extra Ps you might find:

Plan – Another P you might see in the STOPP Technique is "Plan." Plan before you proceed. It works in a similar way to "perspective," but the focus is more on what you're going to do next. *What is the most important thing I can do now?* This is the plan on how you move forward.

Practice – The final P in many therapists' STOPP Technique is "Practice." With any mindfulness technique or coping method, the best thing one can do is practice it over, over and over. This means using the STOPP Method whenever you can, even when you're not feeling anxious, overwhelmed, depressed, sad or lonely. The more you do it, the faster it will become second-nature. Practice it during moments that you usually ruminate, like when making a cup of tea, coffee or brushing your teeth.

This methodology may seem basic, but once you've mastered it, then you'll lean on it time and time again as a management method! The key is *consistency* and to keep practicing, even on the good days. That way, you'll have a viable and valuable tool in your arsenal for the bad days.

Please remember, I am not a professional therapist but I have used these methods and know of many others that have. We have all found them to be beneficial.

As I mentioned before, you are going through this journey to become more self-aware of your emotions and feelings. This is a skill that can be developed and it is well worth the effort to acquire.

Maya Angelou said this: "I've learned that people will forget what you said, people will forget what you did, but people will never forget how you made them feel."

In this case it is ourselves who we're trying to make feel better. It is because of our loss that we feel less loved and we want to regain that lost love. Let's strive to make ourselves emotionally better and we can love ourselves (and others) more and migrate to a better moment in time.

Join me in the next chapter as we talk about just that. TIME! And how it plays a crucial role in our migration and restoration process.

CHAPTER 6

Time Is On My Side! Yes It Is

This Rolling Stones hit has always been a two-edged sword for me. I love the song, released by them in 1964, but when I heard it I always questioned how can time be on your side? Frankly it was its contrary and rebellious framing that probably made it a hit, especially with the social climate of society in the 60s. Probably almost everyone has heard the cliché "beating the clock", so how can time be on our side? Personally I don't think it absolutely can be; however when we wield to the power of Time's confines there is a way to make it work for us.

It is much like putting a harness on a mule, one of the most stubborn animals there are, so that we can harness the mule's power and work ethic. And with that harness we can get the mule to help us prepare our ground for planting, even though he is despising every moment of being our assistant.

So what does time have to do with the grieving/mourning process and the migration to a more functional life? Maybe that sounds silly, but if you're like me sometimes I can get so caught up in thinking, contemplating and self talk that an hour can slip by when it only seemed like minutes. Managing one's time is absolutely key.

As King Solomon said, there is a time for everything. There is a time for focusing on what needs to be done for survival and sustenance. There is a time for relaxing. There is a time for sharing. (Ecclesiastes 3:1-8) There is a time for conversing with friends, and on and on. But more importantly within our thoughts surrounding this book, there is a time for grieving and commemoration.

Yet in all these we need to maintain our focus so our grieving and commemoration don't have a Pac Man effect and eat all our time that needs to be used for other things. As the well-known maxim states, "idle hands are the devils workshop" and the cliché "too much time on my hands" are two places we *do not* want to find ourselves when we are going through the grieving and mourning process.

Thus it brings us to this place where we must manage our time to the maximum, yet still allow for those moments when we need to remember, process, cry and commemorate the loss of our loved one. In this chapter we are going to talk about some tools we can use to put the harness on the mule of time.

Previously, I mentioned my business mentors Matt Robinson and J Paul Mills. There was another book that they recommended shortly after Dylan passed away, "The Miracle Morning: The Not-So-Obvious Secret Guaranteed to Transform Your Life - Before 8 AM," by Hal Elrod. It was the first book they recommend I read.

Soon after J Paul and I were talking. He had just bought a sailboat and he thought it was ironic that I had a model like his boat. I told him I didn't believe in coincidences and then he shared a tingling phrase that his mom used... She didn't believe in *coincidences* either, so she called them *co-incidences*. What a perfect way to describe those ironic, sometimes *deja vu* moments. The reason I mention this is that their book recommendations and my bringing them on as business mentors was perfect timing for what I was experiencing and would continue to experience. Both of those books they recommended have been key elements for my migration to a more functional life without Dylan in this physical realm.

Hal Elrod has an entire community and set of resources for the betterment of people and mindsets. If you've never read his book, you absolutely need to, as in beginning yesterday. You will thank me later. So specifically I want to share with you one portion of Hal's book that has completely transformed my life. It is what he calls the Life S.A.V.E.R.S.

Part 1—The Start Of The Day

Hal recommends you start your day, by spending an hour on this set of transforming rituals. The reason he suggests and recommends this first thing in the morning is that it sets the tone for the day and if one tries to do it later in the day it's usually sidetracked by the whirlwind of things that are going on in the day. And if you don't have 60 minutes there is a six-minute version—or you can create a custom version. By the way as of January 1, 2022 he has now added an app that has the tool you see here. The following is the breakdown of what these tasks/rituals look like.

A sample 60-minute schedule of the Life S.A.V.E.R.S. would look like this:

> **Si**lence (5 minutes)
> **A**ffirmations (5 minutes)
> **V**isualizations (5 minutes)
> **E**xercise (20 minutes)
> **R**eading (20 minutes)
> **S**cribing (5 minutes)

In the six-minute version of this ritual, you spend just one minute on each segment.

Now let's define what each of these segments is designed to encompass.

"Silence is golden" is a term we are all familiar with. When King Solomon was building his temple thousands of years ago, notice what history has to say about the process.

> *⁷ And the house, when it was in building, was built of stone made ready before it was brought thither; so that there was neither hammer nor ax [nor] any tool of iron heard in the house, while it was in building. —*
> *1 Kings 6:7*

A house that he was destined to build that would become a place for silence, meditation and prayer was built in silence with as much intent as possible. Personally that resonates with me as to how important silence is. It is a time when we can have clarity, peace and allow the seeds of vision to spring forth. Hal also suggests that this time can be used for reflection, deep breathing and or gratitude. Again get the book because he delves into each of these segments in far greater depth than I am going to. I just want to create an awareness for you so that you will highly consider making it a habit of your own.

I personally break this section into two sections. I have a minute of silence and a minute of prayer or meditation. It has proven for me to be very powerful to set the tone of the day and create clarity.

Affirmations are everywhere. No matter what religion you investigate, at the core are affirmations. But how important are they? Muhammad Ali (who is vastly recognized as one of the most significant and celebrated sports champions in the 20th century) was hailed as Sportsman of the Century by Sports Illustrated and Sports Personality of the Century by the BBC. This was in in 1999. He lived and breathed his life with quips and quotes that were his personal affirmations. And these words shaped who he was in the minds of those who were familiar with him. I want to list a couple of his quotes/affirmations and then one affirmation that is relative to this subject matter.

> *"Float like a butterfly sting like a bee – his hands can't hit what his eyes can't see."* If you ever saw one of Ali's fights this affirmed who he was in the ring.

"Live every day like it's your last, because someday you're going to be right." This is very apropos in regard to subject matter of this book.

And then finally...

"It's the repetition of affirmations that leads to belief. And once that belief becomes a deep conviction, things begin to happen."

Understanding the connection yet?

This was the epitome of who Mohammad Ali was and who he became. Hal Elrod has several affirmations in his book, within his community on Facebook, and on his website, that may fit with your goals, dreams and aspirations. In the book there is a section that shares how you can create your own affirmations tailored specifically for you. And you may feel you aren't ready for all this, yet it is what one needs to aspire to, so that we can migrate to a more functional self.

Visualizations, simply put, is mental rehearsal. Whether we realize it or not every day, everyone is on stage. Our audience maybe slim and we may not have sold tickets to our performance or get paid royalties, but we are on a stage—the Stage of Life.

Any polished entertainer or celebrity will share that to master the stage, your part has to be emphatically rehearsed. So visualizations are rehearsal of how we want to see our part play out in our mind before we go on stage. This type of mental rehearsal is advocated by a plethora of celebrities and sports figures. And they all attribute their success to visualizations as a key factor.

So to think along these lines let's think of an event or just your day. Imagine and visualize how you emphatically *want* it to materialize. Specifically the best solution would be to consider the day in advance and what plans you have. Then visualize how you want things to play out. You can obviously practice these visualizations before specific events throughout the day, but, my humble suggestion is in the morning start will an overall expectation visualization of the day.

You have the ability to create your own visualizations. Again in his book "Miracle Morning," Hal Elrod provides key thoughts on how to individualize your personal visualizations.

Exercise. I don't think "exercise" requires an explanation why it's a good thing. But maybe why it's good in the morning would be a valid discussion. As I said earlier, exercise makes for a good foundation for the day and sets the tone for the day. Personally I do 52 crunches in my one minute and just that little bit it makes me feel better, more accomplished and gets my proverbial juices flowing. Disclaimer: Maybe I don't need to say this but consulting your doctor may be necessary before beginning an exercise routine, due to health issues you may have.

Reading is fertilizer for the garden of the mind so that our seeds of greatness can grow, and blossom us into who we can become. We become what we read. Personally I read something inspiring, a devotional or a set of passages from the Bible. Whatever you read, look for something that is going to help you grow and assist in your inspiration.

Scribing (AKA journaling) has been "a thing" since letters and writing instruments came into existence. Why would you want to write in a journal every day? I'm glad you asked, as Hal suggests in "Miracle Morning" there are several benefits.

- It helps you elevate to a higher level of gratitude.
- It helps you focus on your wins.
- It helps with clarity so that what needs to change can be addressed.

In the novel "The Leopard," author Giuseppe Tomasi di Lampedusa has Tancredi, one of his characters, make this profound statement:

"If we want things to stay as they are, things will have to change."

Scribing/Journaling provides clarity to see what needs to change. Consider this meaningful quote:

"Writing is the only way I have to explain my own life to myself."

—Pat Conroy, My Reading Life

Hal mentions several other benefits in the book. Have I mentioned that you need to get this book??

Part 2—The Rest Of The Day

Now that we have established a most excellent foundation for every day's beginning, we need to see how we can best manage the rest of the time of the day that is left to our disposal. The very wise Benjamin Franklin said the following:

"If you fail to plan, you are planning to fail"

We will talk more in depth about this in Chapter 9, but in order for us to maximize the time in front us on any given day, we need to have a plan in place. Our plan could include a superfluity of tasks, or goals, or destinations, etc. But whatever it is we want to do to make the most of our time we must plan it out with artistic detail. One of the best ways I have found to do this, is with *time blocking*.

What is time blocking? I know I said this before, but I'm glad you asked. I truly am. If there was a pain pill for taking away the perceived pain (that is embraced by some) of time management, time blocking is that high-potency pill. The *Pomodoro Technique* (AKA Time Blocking) was first developed in the late 1980s by entrepreneur Francesco Cirillo while he was in college. He became frustrated with not being able to accomplish all that he wanted to in a timely manner. At that time he used a timer that looked like a tomato to begin honing and defining the process. In 1992 he introduced what he named the Pomodoro Technique. After reading "Miracle Morning," I began using this methodology and my effectiveness, time management, and feeling of accomplishment skyrocketed.

How does this method work and what does it look like? Let me share with you. You can use what Cirillo found as the primo time frame of a 25 minute block of time to accomplish or strive to accomplish what needs to be done. The following is a list and brief explanation of what this looks like.

Step 1 – Determine What Needs to be Done and the Time Needed

Calculate how much time and effort will be necessary for individual tasks to determine how many pomodoros are needed. If you have short tasks that only takes 5-10 minutes, find similar small tasks that can be batched (properly named task batching) together in one pomodoro. If it's a longer task that will take about an hour, break it up into two pomodoros.

Step 2 – Notate Distractions Versus Letting Them Derail You

Your ability to complete your tasks within any given pomodoro hinges on how well you secure your time blocks. The 25-minute timeframe helps to increase and maintain focus, but you also need a system for handling distractions before they sabotage your progress.

Begin by creating a methodology for handling requests from coworkers, family members and customers. Cirillo suggests using a strategy called "inform, negotiate, schedule, call back." Simply let the person know you're in the midst of something, determine another time to handle their request, schedule a time, then follow up. If a distraction can't be deferred, you'll need to end the pomodoro and start it over from the beginning once the distraction has been addressed. Cirillo also suggests that any time you get distracted you make a note of it. Doing this will help you stay focused on the task at hand and get a better view of what distracts you and how you can continue to improve handling of distractions.

Step 3 – Begin Your First Pomodoro

Along with your list of tasks you want to complete your only other necessity for the Pomodoro Technique is a timer. Cirillo still uses his wind-up pomodoro timer, but you can use the timer on your phone or similar apps such as the Pomodoro timer.

When your timer starts, it can't be stopped. If you stop the timer this essentially nullifies the pomodoro. With the same diligence and discipline, once the timer rings you'll need to stop what you're doing. The Pomodoro technique relies on strict adherence to 25 minutes of intensely hyper-focused work. This is then followed by five minutes of downtime that isn't related to your work.

If the task is finished before the timer runs out, use that extra time to review your accomplishment, make improvements or notes about what you learned, and get ready to move to the next pomodoro.

Step 4 – Expand Your Downtime as More Pomodoros are Completed

When you have completed four back-to-back pomodoros, you need to increase your rest time to 15–30 minutes. Your brain needs more relaxation, resting and chilling after two hours of highly intense super focused work.

Step 5 – Track Your Progress & Analyze Your Efforts

Before going to bed at the end of each day, take some time to review your pomodoros and record your progress. Were your time estimates correct? Did you accomplish what you set out to do? This will help you better determine the effort needed for certain types of tasks so you can improve your pomodoro scheduling.

Also, make note of your productivity each day by tracking your pomodoros in your journal/daily calendar. Make a note of each day that you follow the habit.

Step 6 – Begin Formulating Timetables

Your ultimate goal should be to create accurate timetables for your pomodoros, based on your schedule, distractions and the amount of effort/time that your different tasks require.

The time of day can impact your time blocks. When laying out your pomodoros, notate how you feel and what's happening at different times throughout the day. Those tasks that require the most concentration and mental clarity should be done earlier in the day when you're fresh and are less mentally fatigued. This exercise will assist you in maintaining your pomodoro schedule. It will also keep your productivity at its highest levels.

There are other variations of time blocking, such as *time batching,* which is combining similar tasks. There is also the variation of *Day Theming,* which is defined as using different days of the week for different types of tasks. Personally I prefer the pomodoro time blocking method. It's effective and I get so much accomplished.

Hopefully the relevance of this chapter resonates with you in that it's necessary to stay as busy as possible during this time of grief. I completely understand that sometimes, a smell, a noise, a picture or even something completely obscure causes us to remember our lost loved one. Take the time that's needed to feel how you need to feel and grieve. But try as much as possible not to let it overwhelm you.

Staying busy serves as production but also as a distraction. Maybe you don't work or are unemployed or even disabled. Even with these situations there are many things that you can do, such as volunteering or even doing remote work. Consider any of these things if they can keep you busy.

Join me in the next chapter where we discuss one of the most beneficial ways to assist in our migration and that is in helping others. See ya there!

CHAPTER 7

Help Somebody If You Can

In Chapter 4 I mentioned Ronnie Van Zant. Ronnie has two brothers Johnny and Donnie. Johnny became Skynyrd's new front man after the crash and Donnie has always played with 38 Special. A few years ago they had a duo called Van Zant. They released a couple of albums and on their second album they released a song written by Jeffrey Steele and Kip Raines called "Help Somebody."

I absolutely love this song for many reasons. It's about a reflection of conversations with his grandparents about the things to do to maneuver wisely in this life, and they always end their conversation with "help somebody if you can!"

These lyrics are extremely wise words. In this chapter we are going to discuss how lending a helping hand is not only beneficial for those we help but also how much it *helps us.*

The following illustration speaks volumes:

> **THE LADY**—"Well, I'll give you a dime; not because you deserve it, mind you, but because it pleases me."

THE TRAMP—"Thank you, mum. Couldn't yer make it a quarter an' thoroly enjoy yourself?"

As I write this chapter, we are just a few days past Christmas 2021. Think of the billions of dollars that people spent so they could give gifts to the ones that they love. Doesn't that speak volumes?

Think of how good it makes you feel when you give gifts to those you love and those that you just want to help. Even if it's only for a few moments we are focused on seeing the joy and happiness that our gift brings to someone. And for these moments we experience that ethereal feeling of selflessness. It is that ethereal feeling that can help us set aside our grief for a time.

You know why? Because unfortunately, and this is not a criticism, grief often creates a self-focused, self-absorbing atmosphere that surrounds us. It's natural and the fact is we can get sucked down the drain of life and that is why balance is necessary.

But one thing that seems to be confusing in this help and charity arena is the idea that money is really what you need to be helpful and giving. The truth is sometimes your time and kind words are worth far more than the gold you might be able to spend. There is a saying (we're not sure who coined it) but it goes like this:

People don't care how much you know until they know how much you care.

This care spoken of is *love* and *time investment*. These are two things that many times are hard to come by, and that's why people truly appreciate them when they are given sincerely.

One other song I want to make mention of that I had not heard until the 16th of January 2022. Tammy and I got the opportunity to go see Mavis Staples of the Staple Singers at the 30A Songwriters Festival in Miramar Beach, FL. By the way guess which song she kicked off her show with? You guessed it, Come Go With Me! But she sang another song of theirs that somehow I had missed, entitled, Are You Sure? It is about having this selfless mindset that we are discussing in this chapter. It was ethereal getting to hear it live. Take a read of just these three lines:

> *Are you sure there's nothing you can do?*
> *To help someone worse off than you?*
> *Think before you answer, are you sure?*

It is easy for me to visualize a person like this because my dad, Robert Huffaker, has been one of the best examples of giving of his love and time more than anyone I know. Dad was the elementary principal where we went to school and he was also a minister. From the time when I was about ten or so going forward, Dad would take me and sometimes my sister with him every afternoon to the hospitals to visit the sick. That was 50 years ago. Up until about two years ago he was still going to the hospital three and four times a week to visit the sick. He was 93 years old then.

He has more friends and acquaintances than anyone I know. He is loved and respected because of his selfless sacrifice, of his caring and love for other people. I would venture to say he has given more in time than the richest of philanthropists have given of their money. I share this not only because I am so proud to call him dad but because it is that kind of helping others that can be so healing for us as we maneuver through our grief.

The following is from a book by Allan Luks, *The Healing Power of Doing Good.*

Helpers High: The healing power of helping others

People have known for ages that helping others is good for the soul. A study based on research here in the United States 20 years ago proves it. Allan Luks followed 3,000 male and female volunteers and outlined the positive effects on their bodies and mental health. Helping others:

1. Decreases effects of disease, both psychological and physical.
2. Produces a rush of euphoria (helper's high), and an endorphin release (natural painkillers), followed by calm.
3. Improves stress-related health problems. Reverses depression, gives social contact, decreasing feelings of hostility and isolation. A drop in stress decreases lung constriction, asthma attacks, overeating and ulcers.
4. Enhances joyfulness, emotional resilience, vigor, and reduces the sense of isolation.
5. Decreases intensity and awareness of physical pain.
6. Reduces chronic hostility.

7. Heath benefits and well-being return for hours or days when a good deed is remembered.
8. Increases self-worth, happiness and optimism. Decreases feelings of helplessness and depression.
9. Establishes friendships, love and positive bonds—and these emotions strengthen the immune system.
10. Proves critical to mental health.

Here are a couple of quotes I think are thought provoking and beneficial. Then we will get into the substance of some actions that we can take to help others.

"Constant kindness can accomplish much. As the sun makes ice melt, kindness causes misunderstanding, mistrust, and hostility to evaporate."

—Albert Schweitzer

And sometimes these misappropriated feelings are within us and focused toward ourselves, therefore making kindness an excellent therapy.

"To ease another's heartache is to forget one's own."

—Abraham Lincoln

It is the act of giving and healing that is most helpful. When we give money, it is a good thing, but it is helping at arm's length. You are not necessarily mentally invested in the giving and helping process.

The following is a great list of 23 assorted ways to help others that should provide fodder for ideas on how you could help others:

1. Do you enjoy cooking? Consider baking some cakes or pies and donate them to a local homeless shelter.
2. Consider joining icouldbe.org and becoming a virtual mentor for a teens.
3. Volunteering at a local school is a possible option. Many schools these days are short staffed. And most will welcome community involvement.
4. Can you knit or crochet afghans, scarves, or other handy items? If so, consider donating them to your local senior center.
5. Do you have friends who have young children? If so, offer to babysit. Your friends would probably enjoy a night out. And children can be uplifting to be around.
6. Do you have neighbors who are sick or homebound? Check to see if they need someone to shop for them.
7. Are there crisis hotlines located in your area or one that you can work with remotely? Consider volunteering for a crisis hotline. Here are a couple of examples: https://twloha.com/get-involved/professionally/ and https://samaritanshope.org/get-involved/volunteer-on-the-helpline/
8. Do you know any elderly folks? Consider taking them shopping, to the movies or for a drive.

9. Most libraries have a story hour. Consider volunteering to read at a story hour.
10. Most cities have homeless shelters. Consider putting together some hygiene kits for homeless people—kits that include a toothbrush, toothpaste, deodorant, soap, etc.
11. Consider getting some food for a panhandler. Make conversation with them and let them know there are still people who care and that they have value.
12. Do you like animals? Consider volunteering at your local animal shelter. You might even consider adopting a dog or cat. You might consider becoming a temporary foster parent for an animal while they look for a permanent home.
13. You can send get well cards to children who are hospitalized through cardsforhospitalizedkids.com.
14. Do any of your elderly neighbors need some yard work done? Consider raking, shoveling or cleaning for them.
15. Ever consider donating blood? Your blood could be what saves someone's life.
16. Consider donating a picture that you or you and your child color to ColorASmile.org. They donate the pictures to children.
17. Do you have any skill sets, talents or specialized crafts? Consider offering to do a free one-day workshop at a low-income community center or a women's shelter.
18. Are you an avid reader? Consider teaching someone to read.
19. Do you have books or clothing you don't use or need? Consider donating these things to a local thrift store.

20. Consider sending a card to someone serving in the military through this website amillionthanks.org.
21. Check with your local city or county jails. Sometimes they have or allow prison ministries. Consider volunteering to be a part of those ministries.
22. Many churches have outreach programs. Consider checking with some of your local churches to see if they have any outreach programs that you might be passionate about.
23. Do small acts of service throughout the day—hold the door for people, let someone go in front of you at the grocery store if they have fewer items. Smile.

These are just a few ways to help others, but hopefully as you read this list it will provoke thought on other things you can do. Choose something that you are passionate about and you will reap the tangible and intangible. You will begin to feel and sense the healing of your actions and time investment.

Now follow me into the next chapter where we will explore the healing effects of being part of a community. See ya there!

CHAPTER 8

Community - If You're Ready (Come Go With Me)

"Is it true," asked a student, "that all the people in the world could live in Texas?" "Yes," replied the professor, "if they were friends." And if they were not friends even the world itself is too small."

—The Homilope

Sometimes in our lives our friends list seems very small. But it seems especially true when you lose a child. Because just like there isn't an English word for a parent who loses a child, there are few people who can truly relate to what we have experienced and are experiencing.

This doesn't make us special or entitled but for sure we fall into a different category. This is exactly why a community of like-minded people and those with shared experiences is necessary for our segment of the population. I don't say this because I believe in division but because we need it. We need a support group. And I believe having a community of friends and acquaintances who share the commonality of a lost child is very necessary for our continued migration to a fulfilling life.

What about the title of this chapter and why I chose it? Please let me share. This song was released in 1973 by The Staple Singers, written by Carl Mitchell Hampton, Homer Banks, and Raymond E. Jackson. It was released on the infamous STAX recording label. It is in my top five of all-time favorite songs. I have at times listened to it literally 50 times in a row. The Staples were the Martin Luther Kings of the music world. The majority of their songs promoted love, community, unity and being equal. On the 16th of January, Tammy and I got to see Mavis perform in Miramar Beach and guess what song kicked off the show? You got it this one! The following are a couple of lines from the song that provide the crux of the theme. I encourage you to check out the song in its entirety as it is very uplifting.

> *Love is the only transportation*
> *To where there's total communications*
> *If you're ready come, go with me*

The following is the perfect portrayal of what a near-perfect community would and should be. I say near-perfect because we are human and prone to mistakes. In moving through this chapter, I want to share many of the benefits and the pitfalls of being in a community or grief group that are specific to our scenario. But stay tuned because in Chapter 10 I want to talk about what we can do as a collective group to help establish these groups for ourselves and others.

- **No Shame in Tears** – A grief group/community is a place where it is an understanding and prerequisite that crying is a natural and accepted action. Unfortunately, sometimes society seems to consider tears as a sign of weakness, and even though we may be weak in the moment tears actually help strengthen our resolve.

"There is a sacredness in tears. They are not the mark of weakness, but of power. They speak more eloquently than ten thousand tongues. They are the messengers of overwhelming grief, of deep contrition, and of unspeakable love."

— *Washington Irving*

- **Communication Connection** – As in any relationship, communication is that which connects the resolved to the unresolved. We can't put a puzzle together unless we have all the pieces. Communication allows us the ability to collect all the proverbial pieces to the puzzle. Is it easy all the time? Emphatically heck no! But it is necessary for us to propel to the highest level of our growth and relationships. What communication can provide is friendships, allowance for sharing of ideas (good and bad), quenching of some of the loneliness we are experiencing and in respect to our scenario we can realize there is no "normal."

- **Growth From Our Experience** – A community allows us a clearer path through grief because we can look around and see the successes and failures of experienced people and see how they are progressing through their individual trials. Just as we can react or respond to situations that arise in our day-to-day walk, we can allow our experiences to define or refine us.

- **Grieving Our Way** – Frank Sinatra released his version of "My Way" in 1969 but most likely the most remembered version was Elvis' version, which was released after his death on October 3, 1977. It surpassed the chart placement on Billboard that Frank Sinatra had enjoyed. I mention this song because those two words are the epitome of our grief. Although our grief maybe similar to that of others, our grief in terms of how we experience it, how we deal with it, etc., is going to be different from others. This is very key in understanding when we are in a group or community of those who have experienced a similar loss.

"The reality is that you will grieve forever. You will not 'get over' the loss of a loved one; you will learn to live with it. You will heal and you will rebuild yourself around the loss you have suffered. You will be whole again, but you will never be the same. Nor should you be the same nor would you want to."

— *Elizabeth Kubler-Ross and David Kessler*

- **Becoming More** – A commonality that seems to occur for those that respond vs. react and allow the death loss to refine them is that gratitude becomes front and center in their lives and living in the now is the focus!

It is our hope that no matter what the circumstances, grieving parents can get through the storms of grief and come out on the other side, stronger, more compassionate, and more appreciative of what we all have right now.

- **The Uniqueness of Our Path** – Russell Brunson names the Jones effect as status. And as much as we would like to be like others around us, we are all different to some extent. Death seems to be the alarm clock that "throws us out of the bed"—realizing how much different, how unique we are. Because the reality is we are the only ones who can walk our path to a more fulfilled life. A community will enlighten us more to this fact.

"End? No, the journey doesn't end here. Death is just another path. One that we all must take."

— *J.R. R. Tolkien, The Return of the King*

- **Rising to a Level of Forgiveness** – As we begin to talk with those who have had similar experiences of the death of a child, we realize there is a point where we can choose or not choose forgiving of ourselves and others. At the end of the day what has transpired *cannot* be changed. Rehashing in the mind only cultivates unnecessary pain and heartache. *We have to let go.* That requires forgiveness. Sometimes forgiving ourselves, sometimes others, and sometimes both. There are things that we wanted to do with our loved ones or things that happened or things that were said that we wish we could take back. Unfortunately, not happening... Forgiveness is the only resolution. We must embrace this fact and move forward. No one said it was easy, but it is a necessity if we want to move forward. Being surrounded by friends and like-minded individuals makes this easier.

"We must accept finite disappointment, but never lose infinite hope."

— *Martin Luther King, Jr.*

- **Becoming What We Think** – Remember when we talked about the evolution of feelings to beliefs to convictions? These things mold us into who we are and who we are becoming. That is why it is so critical to keep a pulse on these things and make sure we are doing proper due diligence. The map is not always clear, but we can find where we need to go if we look diligently enough. Having a community of like-minded people who know they need to help each other to evolve and migrate to a more positive place is a necessity. It's almost like trying to sail a large ship without a crew. We need people to help us remember we need to choose positive memories over regret, love over sorrow, forgiveness over anger, and peace over anxiety.

*"When we are no longer able to change a situation,
we are challenged to change ourselves."*

— Viktor Frankl

* **Be Patient?** – When we begin to converse with others who have had similar experiences, we realize that as much as patience may not have been one of our virtues in the past, now it's time to add it to our list of have-tos. We have to realize this process will take time and we can't put unrealistic demands on ourselves or others. And we have to be patient with our family, friends and acquaintances that don't understand.

"Trust that an ending is followed by a beginning"

— Anonymous

* **Dark Shadows are Hidden by Love** – Being part of a community brings us to the realization that although we have lost a dearly beloved, there are still those here in our presence who want and need our love. Spend quality time with all these people, as that love will enrich our lives, because an enlightenment has occurred that shines of love's immediate and in-the-now necessity. Always remember *Love* is an action, not an emotion.

> *"Love is like the wind, you can't see it, but you can feel it."*
>
> — *Nicholas Sparks, A Walk to Remember*

- **Fearless as Warriors Headed to the Front Line** – Being part of a group of folks who have experienced what we have helps us to realize that we most likely have encountered one of the most torrential emotional storms that can be faced and that any other storm of life can be viewed to be as soft as marshmallows. No one says it's enjoyable, but this does become something that we can embrace as factual. With that in mind there should be few things that can occur going forward that should create unmanageable fear for us.

> *"Confront the dark parts of yourself, and work to banish them with illumination and forgiveness. Your willingness to wrestle with your demons will cause your angels to sing."*
>
> — *August Wilson*

> *7 For God hath not given us the spirit of fear, but of power, and of love, and of a sound mind.*
>
> — *2 Timothy 1:7*

I think it is only fair, to set your expectations, to discuss some potential pitfalls of being part of a community. Although they are few and certainly not worthy of not choosing a community, we should discuss them again to set correct expectations. This a short list of those things that you might encounter, but as I mentioned we will talk more about communities in Chapter 10.

1. One's experience could seem overwhelming because our emotions can easily take charge, especially the first few times you engage in the community situation.

2. It can be discouraging, depending on what your expectations are of the group/community, as you might expect to hear that things get easier down the road. That is not necessarily true. The best thing is to be cognizant of your expectations and approach the community with the expectation that you want to take just one piece of goodness away when you leave the meeting. Don't expect a complete and everlasting healing.

3. Don't attend these groups with expecting a therapeutic solution. The people who steer these groups and communities may or may not be trained professionals. If you feel that is what you need, seek the help of a professional.

4. You may get some bad advice. Remember that you will meet all kinds of folks in these groups and for a number of reasons what they suggest that has been helpful and beneficial for them may not be the wisest solution for you or anyone else. Remember to love and be patient, because frankly that is what we need as well.

5. Once again, I redirect you to what I said in the very beginning about beliefs being feelings. We have to understand, embrace and latch on to this concept. The reason is if we don't it so easily allows us to be judgmental, which can completely skew where we need to go, what we need to think, and what we want to be. As smart as we may think we are and as experienced as we may be, we can't know the hearts of those we are surrounded by. Do not embrace the actions of the speeding ticket scenario. If you don't take anything away from this book but this one fact, I promise that you will be a much, much better person.

We covered a lot of things over these last few chapters that I hope you feel will be of benefit to you. But in order to move to the next level, we *must* put a plan in place and take massive action. Join me in the next chapter where we talk about the 40-day plan to get us started down the right path.

CHAPTER 9

Breathe In, Breathe Out...
Move On

On August 29, 2005, Hurricane Katrina obliterated and destroyed much of New Orleans and the Mississippi Gulf Coast. It was a Category 5 hurricane. The highest sustained winds reached 175 mph. It was even stronger than Hurricane Michael that hit Panama City and Mexico Beach in 2018.

I had been working along the Mississippi Gulf Coast for the past 11 years at the time, so I was familiar with the landscape and historical sites that were scattered all along the coast. I knew the personality that cities will always seem to take on.

In my 40 years that I lived on the Gulf Coast, I have experienced many hurricanes and their wrath is unforgiving. Hurricane Katrina was especially full of wrath. This was also a very difficult time for me personally because during the past year I had lost access to my children, Kymber, Dylan and Tyler.

The title above comes from a song performed by Jimmy Buffet, a native of the Gulf Coast himself. He co-wrote the song with Matt Betton, who was a drummer with Jimmy's

Coral Reefer Band for about ten years. After Hurricane Katrina, Buffet released the album "Take the Weather With You." The above song was on this album, and it is specifically referencing Hurricane Katrina. Given my mental state at the time, the song provided me with a lot of comfort, with the perspective that's presented in the song.

Below is a slice of the lyrics. The song starts with him buying a watch from a street vendor that just says "NOW". He goes on to state that people may think that it was a con, yet he explains that the watch is never wrong. The lyrics progress to state that tragedies that don't kill us can very well make us stronger. Below is a slice of the lyrics. When you get a moment listen and absorb what the message of the song is. Then I will explain how this intertwines with our subject matter in this chapter."

Breathe In, Breathe Out, Move On

According to my watch, the time is now
Past is dead and gone
Don't try to shake it, just nod your head

—Songwriters: Jimmy Buffet / Matt Betton

The last six lines provide the outline of the attitude we should strive to have in living our lives daily. The time in front of us, the time we can "control" is now and what is in the past is out of our "control."

Hal Elrod (whom I spoke of at length in Chapter 6) is also a speaker at many events. And at one of his speaking engagements, he introduced on video the concept of "The 5-Minute Rule." (You can find that video here: https://youtu.be/8VDNa4BA0ck.) In this video he presents the concept that when we have negative situations, he says these words:

*"It's okay to be negative when things go wrong,
but not for more than five minutes."*

We can take five minutes, feel however we feel we need to feel, to vent, scream, whatever, etc. but after five minutes forget it and say these three words." **"Can't Change It."** Because the time is "now", and we need to move on.

One other important thought along these lines is the following. Two of sports greatest coaches have been Pat Riley and Lou Holtz. On their teams they had their players wear bracelets with this acronym, W.I.N. This acronym stood for "What's Important Now." Truly that sums it up and the mindset that we should always strive for. It is only what is in front of us in the moment that we can truly enjoy, embrace and work for our good.

In regard to our grieving, I'm *not* suggesting we minimize our thoughts and commemoration of our loved one in a mere five minutes. But it is the attitude of moving on when we can, realizing that we can't change what has happened as much as we may want to. The key, I believe, is not getting lost in the moment and we will talk about that in the Chapter 10, the last chapter of this book. The fact is that we need to have a transformation and/or restoration to a newer version of us that has migrated to a more functional place.

To accomplish anything in an orderly fashion, a plan is needed. That's why in conjunction with this book, *a 40-day plan is available* for separate purchase to help in our restoration to a newer more functional version of ourselves.

Why a 40-day plan you may ask? Well 40 days is deep seated throughout history, dating all the way back to the beginning. The following is just a mere sampling of all the "40" connections. There's a universal understanding the world over that 40 days holds special significance.

The number 40 is found in many cultures and religions throughout time. After you read this list of 40-day events and practices, we will make the correlation with what that number seems to clearly represent.

- Enki was a god in Sumeria. He was sometimes referred to in writing by the numeric ideogram for "40," which seem to refer to his "sacred number."
- Rain fell for "forty days and forty nights" during the Flood recorded in Genesis 7:4.
- Noah waited for forty days after the tops of mountains were seen after the flood, then he released a raven (Genesis 8:5-7).
- In Leviticus 12 the process is laid out where after a woman has a son, she must refrain from touching anything or going into the sanctuary for 40 days until her purification time is over. It was 80 days if she had a daughter. This same process can be found in Chinese

culture. This same type of process is adhered to by those who are Zoroastrian.

- Spies were sent by Moses to explore the land of Canaan (promised to the children of Israel) for forty days (Numbers 13:25).

- The Hebrew people wandered outside of the promised land for forty years due to their lack of faith in believing God could help them conquer the giants in the land of Canaan. This period of years represents the time it takes for a new generation to arise (Numbers 32:13).

- Goliath challenged the Israelites twice a day for forty days before David defeated him, as recorded in 1 Samuel 17:16.

- Moses spent three consecutive periods of "forty days and forty nights" on Mount Sinai:

1. He went up on the seventh day of Sivan, after God gave the Torah to the Jewish people, in order to learn the Torah from God, and came down on the seventeenth day of Tammuz, when he saw the Jews worshiping the Golden Calf and broke the tablets, recorded in Deuteronomy 9:11.

2. He went up on the eighteenth day of Tammuz to beg forgiveness for the people's sin and came down without God's atonement on the twenty-ninth day of Av, recorded in Deuteronomy 9:25.

3. He went up on the first day of Elul and came down on the tenth day of Tishrei, the first Yom Kippur, with God's atonement, recorded in Deuteronomy 10:10.

- A mikvah consists of 40 *se'ah* (approximately 200 U.S. gallons or 760 liters) of water. This is a direct correlation to the practice of baptism recorded all throughout the New Testament. The mikvah was the vessel but also the procedure. It was typically used before a wedding ceremony and both the bride and groom separately would bathe and immerse themselves in the mikvah prior to the wedding ceremony. In the gospels John the Baptist is spoken of and he was baptizing people in the Jordan River. The people weren't questioning the practice as it wasn't a foreign concept.

- The prophet Elijah had to walk 40 days and 40 nights before arriving at Mount Horeb, as recorded in 1 Kings 19:8. He was running in fear of his life and asked GOD to take his life. But it became a time of restoration for Elijah.

- Jonah warned Nineveh that they had "Forty days more, and Nineveh shall be overthrown," as recorded in Jonah 3:4.

- Before his temptation, Jesus fasted for "forty days and forty nights" in the Judean desert, as recorded in Matthew 4:2, Mark 1:13, and Luke 4:2.

- Forty days was the period from the resurrection of Jesus to the ascension of Jesus, as recorded in Acts 1:3. According to Stephen, Moses' life is divided into three 40-year segments, separated by his growing to adulthood, fleeing from Egypt, and his return to lead his people out, as recorded in Acts 7:23,30,36.

- In modern Catholic practice, Lent consists of the 40 days preceding Easter. Sundays are excluded from the count, there are 46 days in total of Lent.

- Similar "40" connections can be found in Islam, Yazidism, Hinduism, Buddhism, Sikhism and funerary customs of other cultures.
- In psychology, researchers have found that personalities can be changed through handwriting exercises over a period of 40 days.
- In physiology, our skin cells on average take 40 days to renew, and our red blood cells start dying from 40 days onwards and sperm count can be increased in 40 days.
- And finally, something that resonates and correlates with our current times. The idea of isolating those who had contagious diseases from the rest of the community was first found in Leviticus 13, when it was specifically speaking about leprosy and what precautions needed to be taken. In the mid 14th century, the plague was spreading like wildfire across Europe. In what is now current day Croatia, in 1377 the Great Council passed a law to establish a *trentino*, a 30-day isolation period. That provided some resolution, and over the next 80 years similar laws were passed in other cities. However eventually the isolation period was extended from 30 days to 40 days, and the name trentino changed to quarantino, a term derived from the Italian word quaranta, which means "forty."

As you review these different 40-day time frames it will likely become very apparent that 40 days is representative of transformation (renewal, repair, regeneration, restoration and rebirth).

So, for this reason with this book there's a 40-day plan that will be expanded to two 40-day timeframes for future use if needed.

Here's a brief explanation of the plan:

- It begins with a dedication page for your loved one.
- The second page will have space for you to note special dates and plans that you have for those special dates.
- There will be a page that will have 40 daily inspiration quotes that will correlate with each day of the plan.
- On the next page (if you want to use it) there will be 40 Bible scriptures that will correlate with each day.
- The next page will be dedicated space for you to write your daily affirmations.
- The next page will have a space at the top for you to check off your daily S.A.V.E.R.S. activities. At the bottom of that page will be space for you to note your time blocks and to-dos during those time blocks.
- On the following page will be space for you to scribe your notes for the day. This will be called **Journal Junction**. It is followed by a space named the **Gratitude Great Room** because it should take a great room for you to list all the things you are grateful for.
- The next section is called **Community Connection**, a place to make notes of your time with your community and accomplishments.
- The next section is for **Healthy Helping**, a place for you to note what helpful things you have done on this day.

- And finally, there's a section called **Commemoration Corner** for you to list anything you did to commemorate your loved one on this day.

I sincerely believe that this will set you on your way to your migration to a more functional place. We are planning to have other activities and solutions to help facilitate this process.

Join me in the next chapter as we wrap up the book and talk about how we need your help to create a community for those of us who have lost a child. I look forward to your ideas, assistance, and all that we can do to support each other in moving forward.

CHAPTER 10

Moving Forward

"Maybe we feel empty because we leave pieces of ourselves in everything we used to love."

— *R. M. Drake*

As I have with many of the chapters, here I have used a song to bring to life the theme of the chapter. This one is no different. Another one of my favorite songs in my top five is the song "Lost In The Moment," written and performed by Edie Brickell. She is the current wife of Paul Simon. This song typifies how we can sometimes feel but to me it also reminds me that I cannot get lost in the moment if I am going to continue to live. The song is about a man who robs a store and, in the process, shoots the store owner. The other characters in the song are the wife of the store owner and their newly born child. It proceeds to share the perspective of each of the characters as the story plays out and what they all need in the present moment that they are in. With the premise of the song being that each one of the characters are lost in the moment of what they need in that moment. When you have a few minutes listen to the entire song to understand the depth of its meaning. The following is a slice of the lyrics as she spells it out so eloquently.

LOST IN THE MOMENT

The tree they planted has started to bloom
She wanted him to see this she wanted him there
She wanted to kiss him and brush back his hair

So, if we don't want to get lost in the moment(s) we must *move forward.*

I need your help, as do those others, those who fall within our commonality of having a lost child. Although there are some groups and resources that I will list in a moment, there aren't physical groups for people—many times even in larger cities—who have encountered what we have. We need that community.

There is no word in the English language that describes the parent who has lost a child. There is a word in ancient Sanskrit that is descriptive. *Vilomah.* It means "against the natural order." So I would like us to collectively come up with a word or phrase that defines us and work toward including it in the English dictionary.

As I mentioned in Chapter 1 the net proceeds of this book are for philanthropic purposes and for us to market and establish virtual and physical support groups. The website is www.lostarrowsbook.com and there will be correlating social media groups to help promote our objectives.

As I mentioned above there *are* some resources available. One such resource that I am part of and have participated in some is a group called *Actively Moving Forward*. They have a very comprehensive app for smart devices. Fran Solomon and her team have done an excellent job in providing a wide array of resources for those that have lost loved ones. I encourage you to download the app and check it out.

Finally, **thank you for taking the time to read this book**. I hope and pray that you have found it helpful and beneficial. And most of all I look forward to connecting with you in one of our portals very soon!